MY SYSTEM

15 Minutes Exercise a Day For Health's Sake

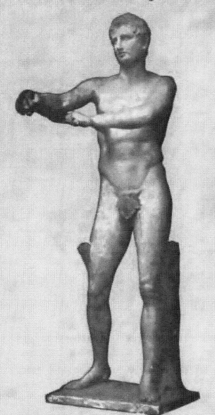

By

Lieut. J.P. MULLER
THREE SHILLINGS & SIXPENCE

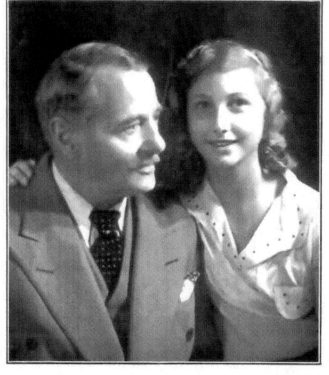

THE LATE AUTHOR, IN HIS 71ST YEAR, WITH HIS GRAND-DAUGHTER,
MIRABELLE, AGED 11½ YEARS

MY SYSTEM

15 Minutes' Exercise a Day for Health's Sake

BY

J. P. MULLER, K.D.

Author of " My System for Ladies," " My System for Children," " My Breathing System," " The Daily Five Minutes," " My Sunbathing and Fresh Air System," etc.

Under the patronage of H.R.H. the Prince of Wales, 1922-1935

NEW EDITION REVISED BY CAPT. I. P. MULLER

WITH 120 ILLUSTRATIONS

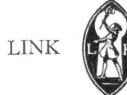

LINK HOUSE

ATHLETIC PUBLICATIONS, LTD.
LINK HOUSE, 24 STORE STREET
LONDON, W.C. 1

A Few Words about Apoxyomenos

The picture on the cover of this book is from a photograph of the antique marble statue, now in the Vatican in Rome, which was found in 1849 in a broken state at Trastévere, near Rome.

Apoxyomenos (Greek—the scraper) represents a young man cleansing himself with a bronze scraper, after athletic exercises, of oil, sweat, and dust. The marble statue is a copy of the bronze statue, well known in ancient times, by the Greek sculptor *Lysippos* (360-316 B.C.).

Much has been written about this statue, but all concur in praising its beauty, and in admiring the Greeks, who, by means of their athletic sports and physical training, were able to produce human forms fit to serve as models for such sculpture.

I have expressly chosen Apoxyomenos from among the many beautiful statues of antiquity to decorate the cover of my book because he is the embodiment of the contents of it : he is the Athlete cleansing and caring for his skin after exercise, and is thus the Ideal towards which my book points.

Under this pseudonym, generally abbreviated to *Apox* or *Ap*, I wrote for a number of years on Athletics in Danish papers.

MADE AND PRINTED IN GREAT BRITAIN BY
THE STANHOPE PRESS LTD,
ROCHESTER : : KENT

CONTENTS

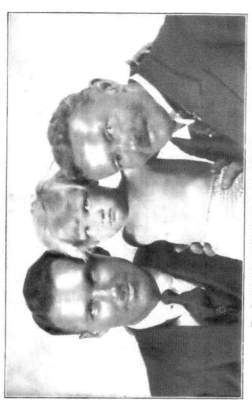

The Author With his First Son and Youngest Granddaughter

INTRODUCTION

It may be of interest to English readers to know a little more than he himself tells us about the person and achievements of the author—who in his own country, Denmark, and in several parts of the World, was a celebrated and justly esteemed Amateur Athlete, Hygienist and Philosopher.

J. P. Muller, who was born in 1866, entered the University in 1884, first studied theology, and then became lieutenant in the Royal Engineers. For ten years he was a private engineer, and for four and a half years Inspector at the Vejlefjord Sanatorium for Consumptives in Jutland, but resigned this appointment in order to devote himself entirely to propagating the cause of Personal Hygiene and completing some important ethical works (not yet published in England).

By means of physical exercises and athletics he developed himself from a delicate boy into one of the most successful all-round amateur sportsmen and athletes on the Continent.

Carl Bloch, the most famous of Danish painters, once said to him : " You are physically the most perfect man I ever saw," and Dr. Krajewski, of St. Petersburg, the " Father " of Athletics, wrote, in a letter : " Really, so splendid a figure as yours, bearing so close a resemblance to the antique statues, is rarely to be met with, either among amateurs or professionals," remarks which are sufficient testimony to the admirable physical development of the man. In this connection it may be noted that the author won in 1904 the first prize at the Athletic Union Physical Culture Competition as the best-developed man in Denmark ; and, after the lecture held in Glasgow on September 19th, 1911, Mr. F. H. Newbery, Principal of the Glasgow School of Art, in proposing a vote of thanks to Lieut. Muller, spoke enthusiastically of the interest and value of the demonstration which had just been witnessed. He had, he said, been for thirty years dealing with living human models ; he had seen Sandow and Hackenschmidt and many others famous for their physique, and hundreds less widely known, but never had he seen in all his experience so beautiful a body as Lieut. Muller's.

The author won altogether 134 prizes, of which 125 have been Championship and First prizes, and only nine Second prizes. These have been won, not in any *one restricted field*, but in almost every possible branch of sport and athletics : sprinting and long-distance running and walking, long jump, rowing, skating, swimming, plunging, throwing the hammer, putting the shot (16 lbs. avoirdupois), throwing the 56-lb. weight, discus-throwing, spear-throwing, wrestling (Græco-Roman style), weight-lifting and tug-of-war, and in the all-round Athletic Championships.

He was also an ardent and skilful boxer, ski runner, and football player, and in spite of his years still held some Danish records.

In 1917, when 51, Mr. Muller put up a veteran's record, in that between Putney and Hammersmith he cycled, ran, walked, paddled, sculled and swam six consecutive half-miles in 29 mins., 19 2-5 secs.

In 1919 H.M. the King of Denmark conferred a knighthood of the Order of the Dannebrog on Mr. Muller, who between 1883 and 1905 had introduced British athletics, field events, new swimming and life-saving methods, etc., until then unknown in his country.

In April, 1924, Mr. Muller stayed for a week at the French Army School of Gymnastics at Joinville, near Paris, where he taught " The Daily Five Minutes " (in all three degrees) to the staff of instructors, who eagerly took the opportunity of learning how to breathe deeply during quick body-movements, and how to relax the muscles properly

In January, 1925, H.R.H. the Prince of Wales most graciously granted his patronage to Mr. Muller in respect of his works and books.

In September, 1924, Mr. Muller had abandoned the institute business, and was thus once more able to devote his whole time to authorship and lecture demonstrations. His tours during 1925-29 on the Continent were of a triumphal character. In Germany he was in 30 big towns invited by the Municipal Health officers to speak and demonstrate in the town halls. The Press quoted freely the following public declaration made by Dr. Mallwitz, physician at the State Academy for Physical Culture and Sport (in Grunewald, near Berlin) : "When Mr. Muller in 1904 published his System, he was a couple of decades in advance of medical science, not only as a physical culturist, but also as an hygienist. Only recently medical science has begun to understand fully his ideas."

In Denmark he was given an almost royal reception ; a gathering of 3,000 people with bands, standards, flowers, speeches and cheers received him at Copenhagen Station. And with signs of the same enthusiasm—only on a smaller scale—he was met in several provincial towns. In Copenhagen he twice lectured in the new Exhibition Hall, each time to an audience of more than 5,000. The first evening, the Social Minister, Borgbjerg, was in the chair, and introduced Mr. Muller with a vivid description of his whole life since their boyhood when they had played and studied together.

In June, 1926, was published in Danish a selection of Mr. Muller's poems, and he was greeted by the greatest living Danish poet, Jeppe Aakjaer, as a prominent colleague. In some of the poems are depicted the beauties of the Chiltern Hills, especially Ashridge Park, Ivinghoe Common, and the old village of Aldbury.

His sixtieth birthday, on the 7th October, 1926, Mr. Muller spent at his Tring home, reading telegrams and letters. But in Copenhagen the Government's paper, as a demonstration of honour to Mr. Muller, arranged a festival in the " Idraetshuset," where 2,500 people gathered. A prologue in verses praising Mr. Muller's work was recited by the poet Aage Hermann, then followed music by a band of 100, songs partly written to Mr. Muller and sung by a choir of 200, a short lecture on " My System " and displays of boxing, wrestling, fencing and gymnastics by the Danish champions, both men and women.

Almost every Danish and German newspaper contained long articles wherein Mr. Muller was praised as the founder of modern physical culture with its appreciation of Fresh Air, Sun, Daily Bath, and Deep Breathing during exercise. And they unanimously state that it is due to him that whole populations now lead a more hygienic life.

His death at the age of 72 was sudden and came as a distinct shock to his host of admirers. Up to the last he remained extraordinarily active and continued to keep himself fit with daily exercise.

Yet, when it is remembered that as a child he was not expected to survive, it is an amazing tribute to his health teachings that he lived as long as he did. He strengthened a weak constitution to such a degree that it gave him an athletic body which he kept actively engaged for more than the three score years and ten for which man is reckoned to be allocated.

THE EDITOR

THE AUTHOR'S PREFACE TO THE NEW EDITION

The Exercises called " My System " were originally selected and composed for the purpose of keeping my comrades of the Copenhagen Rowing Club and myself fit during the " off " season, as regular rowing practice is not possible during winter in Denmark.

Up to this time, the manuals of physical culture in vogue were published with the main object of selling some apparatus (spring dumb-bells, chest-expanders, etc.). On the title page were usually displayed as " authors " the names of famous stage performers, whose biceps or triceps were their chief credentials.

Seeing the splendid results in general health and fitness of my exercises without apparatus, my friends urged me to let them be published. The first Danish edition appeared in 1904, and had an immediate success ; several reprints had to be issued, even in the first few months, and the fame of the little book rapidly spread to other countries.

The subsequent demand for the book has been so great that it has been translated into 24 languages, the sales numbering millions of copies.

One of the main causes of this phenomenal success has been the general and generous support from members of the Medical Profession all over the world. In some countries, Italy, Portugal and Spain, the book and its companion volumes have even been translated by Doctors of Medicine, who asked me for permission to introduce " My System " amongst their countrymen. These doctors (respectively, Dr. Alessandro Clerici, Dr. Ardisson Ferreira, and Dr. Alberto Conradi) put their full names on the title pages and wrote long eulogistic prefaces.

It was the scientific merits of " My System," its recognition of the fundamental importance of the establishment of general health in all the vital, organic functions, rather than in the development of merely muscular strength, which commanded the immediate approval of the Medical Profession.

The endorsement of the " System " by the leading medical men of Europe, the constant comments and favourable analytic reviews in the Continental medical Press, the publicity given to it at several Medical Congresses, where it formed the subject of addresses and debates, and last but not least, the references to it in numerous medical works published by well-known Continental savants, speedily commended it to British physicians, who were only too ready to investigate a physical culture system so free from the taint of commercialism, and which recognised as essential the importance of medical advice in carrying out the instructions.

From 1905 to 1912 I spent my time mainly in travelling in all the countries of Europe, giving lectures and demonstrations ; but in 1912 I gave way to the persuasions of English friends and settled in London, where " The Muller Institute " was established at 45 Dover Street.

The aim of my first editions was first of all to show how the fairly healthy, average person could keep fit, fortify health and stamina and increase physical and mental efficiency. But as so many doctors recommended the book to chronic sufferers and placed it in the hands of their patients, it became more and more evident that this " System " also formed a splendid means of curing several chronic ailments.

This fact has been further proved in the last nine years, during which period a steadily increasing number of doctors have sent their patients to be treated at the Institute. The list of specialists and medical practitioners in London and the suburbs who recommend my exercises to their clients now numbers over 500, of whom 20 are titled, and many Fellows of the Royal College of Physicians and of the Royal College of Surgeons. Several of these doctors have had personal instruction at the Institute for the benefit of their own health, and a number have sent members of their own family.

Several thousand persons have been instructed and treated at the Muller Institute, or by special course sent by post. But the millions, the great mass of the population of the whole Empire are, of course, lacking the opportunity or the means of securing such personal or special attention.

I AM, THEREFORE, PUBLISHING THIS NEW EDITION IN ORDER TO GIVE EVERYBODY IN THE WORLD AN OPPORTUNITY OF BENEFITING BY ALL THE VALUABLE EXPERIENCE GAINED DURING RECENT YEARS.

In former editions only a strenuous form or degree of each exercise was fully described. It was often, therefore, rather risky for patients to do them on their own account, and it was difficult for their medical advisers to explain to them how the same exercises could be done in milder forms. Now, in this new edition, the very easiest degrees or quite simple preliminary movements of every exercise are described in full detail and profusely illustrated. It is further explained which exercises are best for most common chronic diseases or bodily disabilities. The task of the medical adviser who prescribes my exercises is consequently much easier, and his prescriptions are sure to have still more beneficial results than formerly.

People not suffering from any ailment, but who are of advanced age or unaccustomed to physical exercise, can study this new edition, and by following the exercise programme for beginners laid down on page 52, learn the whole " System " properly and correctly.

In the description of each exercise I have warned against every possible mistake which otherwise might have disappointed the hope of deriving good and speedy benefits.

Since the patronage of H.R.H. the Prince of Wales was graciously granted for my works and books and not for institutes, I am no more connected with this line of business.

J. P. MULLER

MY SYSTEM

HEALTH VERSUS ILLNESS

Why be Weakly ?

It has often surprised me that so many people are content to be weak and ill, when in reality there is only a slight effort required on their part for them to grow sound and well, and remain so. But certainly there is a general impression abroad that illness and delicacy are things that must be : a necessary evil.

There are, however, people of both sexes who actually make a parade of their ailments and what they consider to be their " pale and interesting " appearance, under the impression that pallid, sickly looks are an infallible index of an æsthetic and soulful nature. Other signs of ill-health and weakness, such as premature baldness or corpulency, are regarded by many as marks of dignity and distinction—the same false dignity which forbids people, for instance, to indulge in so healthy and beneficial an exercise as running.

Some of our men of letters* have caused incalculable mischief to youth by systematically extolling, both by their example and in their writings, a mixture of exclusively intellectual culture, physical decadence, and mental morbidity. Fortunately there are now signs that their influence is on the wane, so that we who work for the advancement of physical culture, and the moral culture which is its natural result, may also hope for a hearing ; I shall, therefore, henceforward ignore the fact that delicacy of health or appearance is regarded in certain circles as an attribute worth striving for.

Illness is not by any means a thing that one need submit to blindly. Even hereditary tendencies may be successfully combated, and the constitutional inclination held in check.

Antiquated modes of thought are chiefly responsible for the prevailing wrong point of view. Common adages such as " Illness is Everyone's Master !" have made good folk sit down with their hands in their laps, and submit to anything. Many indeed even defy the laws of Nature and the decrees of Hygiene, arguing : " We shall get ill in any case, so let us enjoy ourselves as long as we can ; we need not be afraid that our folly and indolence will arouse contempt ; on the contrary, we shall be objects of gratifying sympathy to the many who think as we do."

If people only knew how much more, how much better and how much longer they can enjoy life if, instead of being controlled by a weakly body, they have a strong and healthy one at their command !

* The English reader must remember throughout that the book has been written by a Dane who is continually referring to Denmark and Danish conditions.

Illness is generally One's Own Fault

Even Hippocrates the celebrated physician of olden times, understood that illness is not a bolt from the blue, but is rather the result of a series of daily small transgressions, which pile themselves up little by little until they burst like a thunder-cloud over the heads of the foolish.

Many people ruin their own health by committing such deadly hygienic sins as always going about in a tight-laced corset and with too high heels, or filling themselves every day with strong drink and too rich and indigestible food, and inhaling and absorbing into their blood, day and night, poisonous gases, which they, and others in the same room, have exhaled and exuded. Many others fall ill through sins of omission. He who does not take care of his body, neglects it, and thereby sins against Nature; *she* knows no forgiveness of sins, but revenges herself with mathematical certainty. If you do not take a bath and some *all-round* exercise daily (a walk does not merit this description), and do not see that you have from seven to eight hours' sleep at night, regularly, it is your own fault if you are ill, for you have troubled neither to get rid of the poisonous matter which is generated in your own body, nor to render the latter capable of resisting infection from without.

It would consequently be absolutely logical to regard it as a species of fraud for persons, for example, who hold business or official appointments, to live in direct opposition to the simplest rules of health, with the result that they are obliged to lie up every year for a longer or shorter period, and entail extra expense upon their employer, the State, or the Municipality, as the case may be, and similarly, if a man be delicate and yet, for the sake of additional profit, saddle himself with more sedentary brain-work, instead of making use of the leisure which his regular daily head-work leaves in order to fortify his health.

Quite recently a man declared in a death announcement that the Government had killed his second child, because there were still not establishments enough for the treatment of poor tuberculosis patients ! There may be *some* truth in the thought, but the State ought in return to have the right to prohibit keeping the sunniest room for show, sleeping at night with closed windows, and without urgent necessity, leading an unhealthy life generally.

We, who make a serious effort to be well, have to watch people committing sins against Hygiene which are simply enough to make one's hair stand on end, without daring, even unobstrusively, to suggest that they should stop. They would certainly retort : " What business is it of yours, Sir ?" Yes, and we have to bear the heavy cost of those places of refuge—hospitals and lunatic asylums—for such " sinners " and their offspring.

Do not point to this man or the other who, despite the fact that he pays no heed to his bodily health, is to all appearance well. His time will come sooner or later. He may possibly be fortunate enough to escape infection, but he will never attain the feeling of exuberant health that a rational care of the body produces. He does not live, he only vegetates. He has wasted the stock of vitality that he may possibly have inherited from healthy parents. His children will be so much the weaker.

So let us not close our eyes, but rather hold up to the light the fact that practically all illness and delicacy is something for which we have to thank ourselves, or at any rate our parents, and let us begin as soon as possible to shake off this yoke of illness, that our children may not when they are grown up, be able to call us to account for allowing them, and even helping them, to neglect their lungs and limbs, and ruin their teeth and stomachs.

What Ought we to Do?

That I have already pointed out. Make use of fresh air and clean water; let the sun shine upon you, and do not let a day pass without every muscle and every organ in your body being set in brisk motion, even if only for a short time. Stagnation in this case, as everywhere else in Nature, is abnormal and leads to drooping and untimely death. Motion is life, increases and maintains vitality up to life's normally late limit.

If illness, pursuant to the law of cause and effect, be as a rule our own fault, we ourselves, on the other hand, can secure the contrary blessings, namely, Health and Beauty. Everyone is the architect of his own happiness; but happiness depends on health, and not on dignities or power, or on a pile of money inherited or scraped together. The business man who, because he has been earning a fortune, has not been able to find time to take care of his health, has doubtless, in many good people's opinion, behaved in an exceedingly sensible manner. But when he comes to reap " the fruits," as they are so well called, of his breathless drudgery, only one of the two following alternatives awaits him: either to die of it all prematurely or to pass the rest of his life in a state of constant annoyance because his poor ill-treated body does not allow him to enjoy life, but compels him to spend his money on specialists or expensive cures. Tacitus of old writes: " *When a man has attained the age of* 30, *he is either an idiot or his own doctor.*" If we put " hygienic adviser " in the place of " doctor," this still holds good. There may of course be cases in which it is judicious to take medicine oneself, or humane to give it to others, but this is an exception and must not become a rule. And in any case everyone ought to know that each time he takes even the smallest dose he increases his distance from the ideal of health, whereas he draws nearer to it by conquering illness *without* the use of medicine—should he happen to have been too late in starting to harden himself against illness. In the same way one ought not always to fly to the doctor for medicine the moment one feels a trifle unwell. (Of course, I am not speaking here about acute illnesses. If you get a serious cold or fever, go to bed at once and send for your doctor. You will then recover in a few days, whereas it may take several weeks if you try to ignore the fever.) One should search in one's own bosom and ask:

" Why am I not so strong and well as I should like to be ?"

The sensible man is obliged to reply:

" I do not trouble to fortify my body in a natural manner; but I will begin to do so now, and thus avoid disease."

If it be stupid to stuff oneself with medicine on the slightest provocation it is simply idiocy to let oneself be led by the nose by all the mercenary, but unscrupulous and irresponsible, business people who through advertisements, with in part, spurious references, prey upon the blind credulity of the public. There does not exist any hocus-pocus, witchcraft, magic cure, or nostrum (such as Gout Tablets, Electric Belts, Elixir of Life, Liver Pills, Nerve Tonics,* or whatever the trash may be called) that is able to give people health. The Philosopher's Stone is nothing of that sort; it is *simply and solely a healthy mode of life*. It is incomprehensible that so straightforward a thing should present difficulties to so many, even among educated and enlightened people. I can only imagine one reason for it—indolence. Of course it is less trouble to take a few pills, a powder, a glass of meat extract, or a draught of elixir, than to exert one's body, even if only for a quarter of an hour. Yes! and it is more refined, more æsthetic, it sounds more aristocratic, to go through a hydropathic cure, than to devote one's attention to these " brutalising " physical exercises.

The cure of disease is the doctor's business, but practical experience teaches that they sometimes regard its *prevention* as beyond their sphere. So we must look after that ourselves. We do not arrange matters here as they do in China, where doctors are paid to *keep* people well. And what is required of us to ensure health is in reality so little, costing a mere trifle in comparison with apothecaries' drugs and patent medicines. The body, so patient under neglect that one often wonders at it, is just as grateful the moment a little attention is paid to it. And when prompt and certain results can be guaranteed and the thing may be done without special apparatus or preparations, is it not worth while to give it a trial?

Some Hints About the Care of the Skin

Even people of the so-called educated classes may be heard to exclaim : " What need to take a bath every day ? One cannot possibly get one's body so dirty if one changes one's linen frequently, and does no dirty work !"

In the first place, I would reply : The loose dirt which comes from without is perhaps blacker, but is not so dangerous as the dirt, consisting of waste matter and poisonous substances, which is given off through the skin in much larger quantities than most people think, and which can be partially absorbed again to poison the body if it be not removed every day. As a proof of the facility with which substances from without can penetrate through the skin to the internal organs, let me mention that if a solution of salicylic acid be rubbed into the skin, salicylic acid can be detected in the urine a few hours later.

And it is not only very injurious to oneself, but very objectionable to those others whose sense of smell has not been blunted by an unhealthy mode of life, to allow perspiration and grease from the skin to stay and putrefy, and be partially reabsorbed by the body. As a rule people are shy of saying such things to one another, but I do not intend to beat about the bush. It is well that people who do not take baths should be told that, even if there be no outwardly visible signs, the fact is patent to one's sense of smell. When such a person has been in my room for one minute—and the windows are always open—I am obliged to have the door open as well, for a time, that the draught may blow the pestilential vapours away. I am not by any means talking of the products

* I have nothing whatever to do with the so-called "Muller Nerve Nutrient."

of respiration, or intestinal gases, but purely and simply of ill-smelling emanations from the skin. And this does not refer only to people of the "working" classes. I have often met "gentlemen" in frock-coats and top-hats, and ladies in evening dress, of whom you could tell by the smell of them, even at a distance of several feet, that they seldom took a bath. It is a special smell, just as people who are addicted to alcohol, for instance, have their peculiar smell. Supposing the person in question to have a bad breath and perhaps be short-sighted as well, so that conversation is regarded as impossible unless the distance between one's face and his be reduced to a few inches, we have an exceedingly disagreeable but uncommonly frequent situation.

In the next place, the bath and the rubbing are intended to serve as skin gymnastics, acting upon the capillary vessels and nerves of the skin, and rendering them sound, healthy, and hardy—which is of the greatest possible importance to the body's general health. One can lay it down as a rule that the good or ill treatment of the skin has an immediate effect on the whole general state of one's health. The skin is not a sort of impermeable covering of the body, but *is in itself one of its most important organs*; we feel with, and partially breathe through it, and we use it to regulate the warmth of our bodies, and to pass off obnoxious matter. It is very beneficial, indeed almost necessary for the health, to perspire a little every day, so long, be it observed, as one washes immediately after. But if there be no immediate opportunity for this, it is essential to keep in movement so as to maintain perspiration until home or some bathing establishment can be reached. How many thousands have contracted pneumonia, or the germs of other diseases, through transgression of this rule! This is especially the case with soldiers, who frequently, after sweat-inducing field exercises and other kinds of exertion, are compelled to remain absolutely inactive for a long time in the cold and wind, or, if it be summer, in the shade, listening to theoretical instruction. A great deal of harm could be avoided in such cases if a dry towel, which could be carried in the knapsack, were passed over the breast and back, even if this were done under the shirt only. It always seems to me to be almost suicidal for a lady heated after dancing, or a perspiring cyclist, to sit down and eat an ice or to drink cold beer. To grow cold while "wet" is always dangerous, whether the moisture be caused by perspiration, rain, or by falling into water with one's clothes on. During evaporation a very large amount of warmth is drawn from the body, and this has the worse effect for the very reason, especially when the moisture proceeds from perspiration, that the process of cooling is very unequal. To be "dry-cold," on the other hand, is not so dangerous; yet it is exactly this of which people have such a horror, and this is why they pack themselves into so many clothes that they break out into perspiration with every little movement, the consequence being that they catch cold at once. People take cold very frequently, not because they are insufficiently clad, but because they wear too many and too thick articles of apparel. It is far less dangerous when stripped to take sun-baths in the open air during the cold seasons; yet this again is regarded as terribly imprudent, so perverse is the public mind regarding such matters.

I have often heard people, even sportsmen and athletes, boast that they could do this, that and the other, without getting into a perspiration; some indeed were so "strong" that they could not perspire at all.

They were proud of what was very much to their disgrace. The pores of their skin were choked with clotted grease and dirt until they could not perspire, while their muddy complexions or flabby appearance were infallible signs of their unwholesome condition.

If the functions of the skin are wholly interrupted, death will ensue in the course of a few hours. Who does not know the story of the little child who was to represent the Golden Age in a procession at the accession of Pope Leo X, and had its whole body gilded over ? A few hours afterwards it breathed its last in convulsions.

It is very right and proper to be in a perspiration before one takes a bath, but the respiration, and, especially, the pulsation of the heart should have become normal again. With regard to the heart, it is of the very greatest importance that breathing be never neglected ; not for one moment must the breath be held during the performance of any exercises, but it must be inhaled and exhaled deeply, quietly, and uninterruptedly through the nose all the time. It is absolutely necessary that the air one breathes should be good. Consequently, if exercises are to be performed in the morning in the bedroom, immediately on springing out of bed, the latter should be covered up again as quickly as possible (of course to be properly aired later on), and then the exercises may be done, provided the windows have been open all night. If not, they must be performed in another room, the window of which has been open during the night. I can, however, hardly believe that anyone who takes the least interest in his or her health would sleep without giving free circulation to the fresh air through open windows.

If afraid of not being warm enough at night, during the winter, it is very much better to put more clothes on the bed, or warmer night-garments on, than to close the window. *The air you inhale can, and should, be cool and fresh.*

A very practical mode of procedure—just as effective, but considerably cheaper than a Turkish or Finnish bath—is to run or walk quickly home from work, so as to get into a heavy perspiration, then take a bath at once, and perform some rubbing exercises, before dressing again for the midday or evening meal. You must of course put other clothes on, at any rate, other underclothing. Let me, at the same time, call attention to the fact that it is an unhealthy and uncomfortable habit to wear the same underclothing night and day ; what is worn during the night ought to hang up to air during the day-time. When hardened you might find it pleasanter to lie quite unclothed in bed, at all events in the summer. For long enough I took no other exercise than the above-mentioned run home, with a bath and rubbing exercises afterwards, and yet kept in splendid condition. And no one can say that it cost either time or money, as I got home more quickly than by 'bus, and saved my money.

No one ought to take a cold bath unless comfortably warm. The more one is perspiring, the colder one can bear the bath, and the more enjoyable it will be. But if one be feeling cold, and for any reason cannot restore the circulation, the bath should be warm.

When, during the summer, it is possible to bathe out of doors, the daily exercises can be performed at the bathing place. After a fairly long swim, if cold, rubbing exercises will be the best means of restoring the circulation. It is a very good plan to undress at once ; in the sunshine especially, you do not want to keep your clothes on for the exercises preceding the bath. People who cannot stand a bright sun on their heads should wear a straw hat or a white handkerchief as a protection. As a general thing, you should let the sun shine on your body (not forgetting the back) whenever you have the chance. By so doing you lay up a store of health for yourself that you can draw upon in the gloomy season of the year. The ancient Greeks well knew how to appreciate sunshine as a health-giver, and, indeed, looked with contempt on a man with a white, spongy skin. Later on, like so much other valuable knowledge, this sank into oblivion until rediscovered by Arnold Rikli* and Professor Finsen.† But there are still only comparatively few who properly appreciate the health-giving properties of the sun's rays. Even in hospitals, where people go to be made well, the blinds are drawn down to keep out the sun even in the winter months, when it shows itself so sparingly, and is so badly wanted ; but those who treat it with contempt do not escape unpunished ! As it is the rays of light, and not the heat of the sun, which have such a beneficial effect on the skin, and through it on the health of the whole body, we can derive great advantage in the summer, even early in the morning, from a sunbath of half an hour, which most people can manage to secure by getting up a little earlier. To make up for this we ought to provide for somewhat more sleep during the dark season of the year. We shall only be adapting our habits a little to Nature's own teaching. Babies, too, derive an extraordinary amount of benefit from crawling about, or playing, without clothes on, in the sunshine, or in warm weather. On the other hand, it is a quite mistaken method of " hardening " children to let them go bare-legged during the cold seasons. It tends, rather, to hinder the growth of the legs. Head-coverings, however, are superfluous for children in almost all weathers, and grown-up people, too, ought to accustom themselves to going about bare-headed. This is the best way of avoiding baldness and nervous headaches, and one comes by degrees to regard the much dreaded " draught " as a morbid superstition. By the way, all these subjects are treated much more fully in " My Sunbathing and Fresh Air System."

The Importance of Relaxation

Whereas the most important principle in exercise is to breathe fully and regularly during all sorts of movements, the next in importance is to relax all those muscles which are not absolutely necessary to the intended performance.

Those persons who understand these two rules will enjoy the everlasting benefit of quick and enduring muscles, with elastic, strong and active organs.

A saying such as " . . . With all muscles taut and the breath held," used in so many novels about men and beasts who are on the point of effecting a coup, has done a great deal of harm by giving the public false ideas. All nerves and senses must, of course, be on the " qui vive " in such circumstances ; but if the muscles be contracted and stiffened,

---

* Arnold Rikli (died 1906), of Switzerland, who established light, air, and sun-baths in the year 1859.
† Professor Finsen, of Copenhagen (died 24th Sept., 1904), discovered the modern system of Light Therapeutics, and treated lupus and other skin diseases in his Light Hospital with great success. He was awarded the Nobel Prize in 1903.

they will *not* immediately obey the nerves' command, and they are tired before having commenced their real work.

Moreover, if the breath is held simultaneously with the tension of the muscles, the result is that the person will be out of breath, and will miss his target or be defeated in the struggle. A champion boxer or wrestler understands to loosen and relax his muscles whilst dancing round his opponent ; and even at close quarters, or in an embrace, it is unnecessary to protect more than one or two points by contracting a muscle. The crawl-swimmer does not last long unless he understands to relax the arm muscles while bringing the disengaged arm forward above the water.

Also the leg muscles, when they have performed the kick or " beat," should be dragged along absolutely slack and relaxed. On the contrary, a so-called " gymnast " or a " strong man " is usually stiff as wood in the arm, abdominal and respiratory muscles, and is, therefore, of no use in any branch of athletics or games whatsoever.

I consider it to be the worst fault of all to maintain the " crampy ' position of "attention" during the performance of my exercises ; also the very much advertised, but really fearfully unhealthy " gymnastic form." I demand that every second moment, namely, during every exhalation, one should " relax " many muscles and " collapse," as it were, as only in this way is it possible to maintain elasticity in all parts of the frame, organs and muscles.

The majority of people, including all " good gymnasts " and bad athletes, age much too quickly, get stiff and short-winded, just because they have never learnt the art, or got the habit of breathing with the whole of the lungs, and relaxing their muscles in time. Even when they are dozing in a " comfy " arm-chair, yes, even when they are asleep in their beds, and are supposed to be resting the whole body, they still have several muscles partly contracted.

The Immediate Effects of Rational Physical Exercise

After a few weeks' work, you will note with agreeable surprise that the fat round your waist and abdomen is beginning to yield place to firm muscles, and, indeed, what I might call a " muscular corset " is gradually developed ; the basis of a strong and healthy body. In women, moreover, this corset will bring about the conditions necessary for painless delivery in childbirth, together with other desirable results. What these " Corset Exercises " also to a very high degree tend to promote in those who practise them are : a good carriage, a straight, erect back, and elasticity and suppleness in all the movements of the trunk.

The entire body is strengthened, and grows flexible, mobile, and efficient. After you have once really become strong all over, as a matter of course you are healthy as well, and if healthy, at the same time—but only then—really beautiful. This is true of both men and women. Beauty is thus identical with health and strength—not a sign, but an expression of it. It can be proved, both amongst human beings and the higher animals, that the shapes and proportions which render the body most serviceable in every respect are the most beautiful and the most harmonious. I am not alluding to beauty of feature or unnecessary strength of arm. Of what use can it be for a chain to have certain tremendously strong links if others are fragile ? One must admit that it is an altogether erroneous mode of speech to call a man strong just because the muscles of his arms are unusually powerful, while perhaps the sources of his vitality—the muscles round his body and his internal organs—are weak. It may in fact be positively dangerous to the health to be much stronger in some of the limbs than in others, or than in the rest of the body. It induces one to overestimate one's capacities. Strains through lifting, stitch, rupture, and nearly every over-exertion of such organs as the heart, arise from this cause. It is as though, trusting to the strong links in the chain, one were to hang upon it as much as it would be able to bear were the entire chain of the same quality. The result naturally is that one of the weaker links gives way, and then the entire chain is broken. Not only have the strong links been of no use, but they have done a great deal of harm by creating a false impression.

But the idea of " strength " has been so much misunderstood, and the word so much misused, that people do not care to do anything in order to become really strong. They have seen again and again so-called strong men hampered by every kind of illness, and often dying at a comparatively early age. And the same with beauty. The erroneous conception that this depends on the contour of the face, the colour of the eyes, the luxuriance of the hair—things which it is not easy permanently to alter—has resulted in people overlooking the beauty that is *bona fide* and valuable, and which, moreover, it is in everyone's power to secure for himself. And yet a fresh complexion, clear eyes, and a free carriage of the head—all of which are the outcome of a rational care of the body—lend a certain beauty to the most irregular features. By following out " My System," and now and again going for a run (on the balls of the feet), you will not only attain perfect health, but the shape and appearance of your body will approach more nearly every day to the ancient classical ideal of beauty, for the simple reason that this coincides exactly with the highest ideal of bodily health, flexibility, and all-round efficiency. And running is not for boys and men only ; women, and especially young girls, ought certainly also to practise running long stretches of sportsmanlike style. Then by degrees we shall be spared the sight of a walking sylph who absolutely must catch her train suddenly transforming herself into a cow or waddling duck.

The art critics of our day, in their remarks anent the classical statues of olden times, have certainly confused cause and effect, probably because they themselves are rather students than practical athletes, and therefore lack the qualifications necessary to understand what colossal and yet delicately and harmoniously balanced physical powers and what a mighty exuberance of strength are represented by a Dory-phoros or an Apoxyomenos, and what a tremendous and unswerving labour must needs have preceded such a result. To imagine that it was love of beauty that produced such shapes and lines is simply absurd. The large capacious chest so characteristic of all antique statues is synonymous with the highest possible degree of strength and endurance in lungs and heart. The powerful oblique muscles of the abdomen, which form the most beautiful part of the celebrated antique torso—a glaring contrast to the thin, unmuscular waists of our present-day athletes—are developed by the very exercises that I have cited later as most strengthening to the digestion and the *intestinal* functions. There are other muscles, as for instance the triceps (on the outside of the upper arm) and the trapezius (at the back and sides of the neck), which are often exaggeratedly developed in present-day athletes, whereas they are never strikingly conspicuous among the ancients. They play no considerable *role* as regards the health or general efficiency of the body, which is the reason I have not laid much stress upon them in " My System."

The chief value and title to esteem of classical sculpture is that it has created models we can admire, learn from, and seek to imitate.

Forty-five Years' Experience

Exercise of every organ and muscle and a bath which is not to cost much money or time or trouble can only be had within the sphere of one's own home. The blessings of home gymnastics are therefore accessible to each and every one who only cares to hold out his hands for them.

Let me tell a little about myself. My father suffered from different bodily infirmities, and when I was born I only weighed $3\frac{1}{2}$ lbs.,* and could be placed in an ordinary cigar box. When I was two I nearly died of dysentry ; as I grew older I contracted every childish complaint, and in my early schooldays I was always ill some few times in the year (with feverish colds, diarrhœa, etc.). I consequently neither inherited my present health and strength nor laid the foundations of it in my childhood. They are qualities acquired through physical exercises, which have been carried out on a plan which has been, year by year, more carefully thought out. Of course, I should have attained this good result much more quickly and easily had I set about the matter at first with the knowledge and experience I now possess. But for that reason I regard it as my duty to render the work easier for those who are striving towards the same goal, but have not yet attained it.

In 1874, when I was eight years old, I got hold of some books translated from the English and German on *The Principle Teachings of Physiology* (Dr. A. Combe) and on *Health Gymnastics* (Dr. Schreber), and I began to do a few exercises on my own account both with and without dumb-bells. A short notice on " Pedestrianism " in *Über Land und Meer* in 1880 taught me amongst other things to run on the balls of the feet, and was the first step towards my being able later—after having studied *Victor Silberer†* in 1885—to introduce walking and running sports on rational lines into Denmark. In 1881 I studied a short popular *Guide to the Care of the Health*, by Trautner, District Medical Officer of Health.‡

I tried, one after the other, every system of Home Gymnastics that came out, and in addition, as years went by, gained considerable experience by practising Gymnastics (partly private and partly club practice), now according to the " Danish " method and now according to the " Swedish," as well as all kinds of out-of-door sports. Still, it

* Danish, very nearly equivalent to 4 lbs. English.
† Austrian author and " father " of sports.
‡ Trautner, " *Vejledning i Sundhedspleje*," 3rd ed. Copenhagen, 1894. (1st ed. 1881.)

was chiefly my private home gymnastics and running in the open air that transformed me from a delicate boy into a strong young man.

My first free and dumb-bell exercises were anything but systematic. Later on I tried various real *systems* requiring to be performed with weights hanging from a cord worked by a pulley. These apparatus were comparatively difficult to set up, noisy to use, and quickly got out of order. Excellent exercises for the development of the muscles could be performed with their help, but no heed was paid to the well-being of the equally important internal organs, apart from the fact that it generally took quite an hour to go through all the exercises. The same objections hold against many English, American, and German sets of apparatus and the systems appertaining thereto, the principle of which is similar, though the resistance produced by stretching an elastic band is substituted for the weights. These bands, however, soon grow slack and are easily broken, so that the necessary apparatus is dear in the long run. My later experience is that all such apparatus tend to stiffen the chest by developing its covering muscles instead of those by which it is actually moved.

I know not a few men who have very strong arms, shoulders and pectorals, but unwholesome blood, and delicate lungs and stomachs. It is of more importance to have vigorous lungs and heart, a healthy skin, powerful digestion, and sound kidneys and liver—quite apart from the fact that it is unsightly for the arms to be proportionately more developed than the rest of the body.

I am, on the whole, opposed to the great *mental concentration* upon special single muscles advocated by so many psycho-physiological systems, as they are called in the advertisements—a half-mystical and alluring name, with a scientific sound. The 15 or 20 minutes a day of home gymnastics ought to be a recreation for the brain, not a fresh addition to the headwork which is already, without it, too great a strain on the average man of to-day.

Some home-systems advocate "stationary running." As I was Danish champion over all middle and long distances, there is doubtless no one who will refuse to admit that I thoroughly understand and am fond of running (the primary exercise of classic times), but as a part of indoor gymnastics, it should not be introduced in any form whatever. If the running be gentle, it loses its chief value as a gymnastic exercise ; if it be violent, the air of the room is set in motion, and the dust whirled up and absorbed during one's forced respiration. Besides which, there is no sense in using up any of the short and precious minutes of our Home Gymnastics in performing *badly* an exercise which one has an opportunity—for instance, on returning from one's daily work—of performing well in the open.

Before concluding this chapter, I must likewise mention the numerous " inventors " of " secret " home gymnastic systems who have sprung up of late years. These are not accessible to the public in cheap books, but, by the aid of puffing advertisements, people are induced to pay exorbitant prices for information as to the exercises. As the latter are drawn up on old familiar principles, they are generally of some benefit, and of course there are always people who are attracted by the mysterious, and who imagine that so long as a thing is thoroughly expensive, it must necessarily be excellent as well.

What I understand by Exercise, Athletic Sports and Physical Culture

By *Exercise* I understand *every kind* of bodily exercise. By *Athletic Sports* I understand movements and exercises which are performed for pleasure or amusement, in order to enable one to excel others in any special branch, or to win in competitions. By *Physical Culture* I understand work performed with the *conscious* intention of perfecting the body, mind, and soul, and increasing one's individual health, strength, speed, staying power, agility, suppleness, courage, self-command, presence of mind, and social disposition. Strictly speaking, one and the same exercise can, subjectively regarded, be sport at one time and gymnastics or physical culture at another. A man who sits in a boat and rows, to strengthen his lungs and the muscles of his back, is performing a physical culture exercise, whereas it is, more often than not, *sport* for a so-called gymnast to vault the horse as high as he can manage, or even for him to strive to make the descent in a high jump as faultlessly as possible. Further, when a teacher of gymnastics tries to get his team to perform free exercises as nearly together as possible, so that they may be able to do better than other teams with which they are to be matched, even when there is no prize nor public mention in prospect, *that* is often only sport too. If, after a completed course of physical exercises, the question asked be : " What can the pupils do ?" the thing is *sport*, but if it be : " How are they now physically ?" then it is Physical Culture.

The moment bodily exercises are chosen in such wise that they tend to the improvement and development of the individual in just those particular points in which he is deficient, they are *rational Physical Culture*. It ensues from this that a system of gymnastics, wrongly applied, may prove in the highest degree *irrational* for the individual, even if ever so rational in theoretical form. For anæmic boys or girls, skin rubbing, sun baths, and deep breathing will be a more rational form of Physical Culture than exercises in a drill-hall, even according to Father Ling's system.*

Physical Culture exercises can only be rational in their application when they take into consideration the needs of the individual. For that reason, team exercises and school-drill can never be more than approximately rational, and, carried on as they are in most cases now-adays, they are anything but that.

If the above-mentioned rower's comparatively weakest points were his lungs and back, his rowing might very well be rational Physical Culture. When a man, in a " Weight-lifting " Club, holds up an iron ball in the air for the sake of beating the existing record, that is Sport ; if he do so for the sake of developing his extensors, it is Physical Culture, and if it be his arms, and in particular the triceps which are comparatively weak, *it is conceivable* that he is performing rational Physical Culture exercises. Still, I have never seen any man or woman whose arms were weak in comparison with their skin, or their abdominal muscles.

For forty-five years I have used my eyes and thought about these things, and I have come to the conclusion that those parts of the human

*Ling, the founder of Swedish Drill and Gymnastics (1776-1839.)

body which in the majority of cases are farthest removed from ideal health and perfection of form are the lungs, the skin and the middle of the trunk, for which reason deep breathing, skin gymnastics and exercise of the muscles about the waist are what nine people out of every ten stand most in need of. A system of gymnastics, paying requisite attention to these points, will have a good chance of being rational, especially in its practical application as Health Culture in the Home.

A quarter of an hour daily is a very limited time, but when it is used to the best advantage it is, nevertheless, sufficient to prevent illness and preserve health, indeed in many cases regain it so that the body is little by little transformed from a fidgety, hypochondriacal master to an efficient and obedient servant. If you will concentrate your attention for fifteen minutes on working for your health, you will get so far that in the remaining 1,425 minutes of the day you need not think of it at all. It is the very people who assert that corporal matters ought not to occupy one's thoughts, whom one always hears talking about their nerves, bad digestion, tiredness, and every imaginable kind of physical disability. Only read one of the many patent medicine advertisements that of Pink Pills for instance, and you will see drawn up a choice of the ills lying in wait for those who will not take a little rational exercise every day—of course, I do not mean that they ought to take the pills!

THE MINOR SOURCES OF HEALTH

What I have hitherto recommended and included in " My System ' in these pages, namely *lung, skin,* and *muscular gymnastics* in conjunction with *fresh air, sunlight,* and *water,* are *the main sources* of health. If they be drawn upon daily, less attention can be devoted to the minor sources. Although they have no place within the fifteen minutes' limit, I will nevertheless briefly state my own experience with regard to them.

Suitable Diet

There are more people who slowly eat themselves to death than there are who die of hunger. So do not always eat as much as you thin you can stuff into you, especially at night, and do not believe that your hunger is always real ; the feeling may be due to some fermentation in the stoma h. A great deal of the food will probably pass through undigested. This wears out your digestive organs before their time. You can see from this how foolish the wise man's words were when he said : " A man is what he eats." They ought rather to run : " What a man is depends on *how* he eats," or " how he digests."

Leave off bolting your food ; do not wash every mouthful down with a drink ; and leave off reading the newspaper at meal-times, thus forgetting to masticate properly. Still you must not fancy that you can live to be eighty simply by chewing every mouthful thirty-six times. If you feel unwell, it will most often be because your stomach is overloaded, and in that case you will feel better for skipping a meal, or for fasting for a day and drinking nothing but water. The plainest meal will then taste delicious.

When your digestion has been invigorated through physical exercise you can safely eat almost every kind of food, but avoid vinegar, strong spices, and condiments, and remember that wholemeal bread, vegetables and fruit, give one more strength and less gout than roast meat and beef-steak. People who eat too much meat often suffer from tainted breath. How often have I not seen digesting the so-called " boat-race steaks" exhaust a crew to such an extent that they came in far behind us others, who had only eaten porridge with milk and rye bread with butter. I have seen big, strong Italians, whose fare consisted only of dry French rolls and thin coffee, work much harder and with greater endurance than, for instance, the Danish workmen, who are fed on meat and strong beer.

Richly prepared meat, highly seasoned dishes, food with vinegar (such as beetroot), sardines, lobsters, strong cheese, and so forth are poison to the stomachs of young people under sixteen. The same applies to such drinks as wine, strong beer, coffee and tea. Even grown-up people would do well to remember that " *strong drink makes weak men.*" But I am not a faddist. I believe in eating and drinking anything in *moderation*, because with a reasonable amount of good exercise the digestion is so enormously improved that one need not worry about what to eat and drink. A glass of beer or wine with meals cannot do much harm, but *everyone* who takes plenty of concentrated spirits daily ought to know that he is breaking down his health by so doing, and in any case his power of resisting disease.

Of the importance of a daily, regular evacuation of the bowels, I need not say much. I should first like to know whether anyone who goes through "My System" every day will be able to wait much more than twenty-four hours. Immediately after rising in the morning, just before going to bed at night, and perhaps also once in the course of the day, preferably midway between two meal-times, a glass of fresh, clean water ought to be drunk. In this way, the intestines, and especially the kidneys, receive a wholesome bath. Hard workers should take three meals a day, easy workers only two.

Sensible Underclothing

A generation ago most boys and young men went about without wool underclothing, according to the comparatively healthier practice of their fathers. Then thick, tight woollen under-vests won their way into favour and contributed considerably to the present generation's susceptibility to cold. I, too, wore wool for a number of years and tried Jaeger's normal clothing for a long time, but I gained nothing by it except that I made myself tender and nearly always had a cold or cough.

When some years later I flung my woollen underclothing aside, my appetite was for a long time twice as large, because metabolism—the waste and renewal of bodily tissue—is impeded by unduly warm clothing. As a matter of course, woollen underclothing ought not to be left off without some previous hardening of the system by means of the daily bath and rubbing. After having made use of my rubbing system for some time, you will find that you do not feel the cold so easily, and will yourself find tight woollen underclothes uncomfortable.

I think the best plan is to vary the underclothing according to the seasons, in order not to feel chilly in winter, or perspire in summer as soon as we walk a little. It is not pleasant to perspire freely unless we mean to do it, during strenuous exercise, when we have changed our everyday clothes for a practical costume. The hardened man should not need more than one layer of underwear, viz., a shirt and pants of a material, varying, according to the temperature, from thin linen or cotton mesh in the warmest summer to thick silk or flannel in the damp cold of the English winter. No undervest need be worn except when wearing a starched front with evening dress.

The healthiest and most comfortable thing for people working in the open air, such as bricklayers and agricultural labourers, would be to wear no clothes at all at their work in summer-time save short knee-breeches, and to put on their coats only when they went home from their day's work. If wrestlers in a circus can show themselves bare to the waist, there will surely be no one who would forbid workmen doing the same for their health's sake. It ought to be tried. In fifty years time it will be universal anyhow, why wait ? Better far to make short work of it and at once abandon the thick, ugly, woollen vest, heavy with putrefied grease from the skin and saturated with stale, evil-smelling perspiration ! I have often in times gone by, when on long rowing excursions in the Sound, got the whole crew to take off their rowing vests. The wind might blow, and we might sweat, but it was only to our own comfort and advantage.

In addition, everything should be avoided that is in any way confining, such as tightly buttoned wrist-bands or neck-bands, tight collars, and garters. Even apparently loose elastic garters can injure the legs by producing varicose veins. It was the fashion once among the Copenhagen street-boys to put a small, thin elastic ring round dogs' tails. The victims felt nothing at first, and their owners also failed to notice the narrow band. But by degrees the tail shrivelled up and fell off.

Moderate Indoor Temperature

What are we coming to ? In times gone by, nobody thought of heating bedrooms or churches ; now we shall soon be having heating apparatus in trams and cabs. Anything over 60° F. is not only not beneficial, but in the long run injurious, in a sitting-room. The body becomes a hot-house plant with no power of resistance. It is easy to accustom oneself to a low temperature. In our office it is never more than 53° to 55° F. in the winter ;* even the lady book-keeper finds it comfortable.

I do not mean, of course, that less fuel should be burnt, but that there should be a window open, at least a little way, the whole time. Warm air that is fresh is naturally better than cold that is bad, and there cannot be sufficient ventilation without warming a room to some extent. To keep in the heat by shutting the windows costs less in firewood but more in *medicine*, which is dearer.

Proper Care of Teeth, Mouth, Throat, and Hair

It does not do to demand impossibilities of busy men, such, for instance, as that the teeth should be brushed after every meal, but bits of meat and the like should preferably be removed with a wooden toothpick.

The following may be regarded as the minimum that can entitle one to be called cleanly and sensible. Brush the teeth and gums up and down, as well as across, and do not forget to brush them inside, at least once a day, and at night very much rather than in the morning, when one might be satisfied with rinsing the mouth out and gargling the throat a few times with warm water containing a teaspoonful of salt. Let some relative (or better a dentist) look carefully at your teeth a few times in the year, to see whether there is any decay. If so, the tooth should be stopped at once ; it pays in the long run.

Do not allow children to eat every day sweets, chocolates, or cakes with sugar upon them, and never hot, or cold, but tepid food. It is not enough to taste it oneself to see whether food is cool enough not to burn ; remember that a civilised tongue and palate are, so to speak, copper-plated.

* This chapter was written several years ago, when I was an inspector at the Vejlefjord Sanatorium. It is quite possible to be content with such low temperature when living in a dry climate. But if the air is moist, the cold is felt more, and a higher indoor temperature will then, of course, be necessary.

The hair must be thoroughly combed and brushed every day, and exposed as often as possible to the invigorating action of sun, wind, and rain. All artificial hair tonics and restorers are indifferent or even injurious.

Some Attention to the Feet

A badly tended foot has something corpse-like about it. But the prevalent opinion is that so long as a sepulchre is well whited, the surrounding world's sense of sight and smell will not be offended by the corpse. As a rule one may assume that the more elegant the cut of the shoe, the uglier and the more deformed the foot itself will be, whether that of a lady or a gentleman. Many people who seldom wash their bodies or their feet would not venture to show themselves in the street without their coat being brushed and their footgear polished, and regard it as absolutely necessary to put on a clean collar every day. Indeed I positively believe that by many people, even in " intelligent " circles, it is looked upon as natural and usual for the feet to be dirty, whereas the hands, of course, must always be spotlessly clean. Otherwise I cannot explain the following instances of, let us say, naïveté. I once overheard a fragment of a conversation between two female school teachers : "Just fancy, his hands were as black as—oh ! what shall I say ?—yes, as *my feet* !" And at a swimming competition at the Royal Docks in Copenhagen, I saw a " gentleman " who was going to take part in one of the races walking about among the company with a student's cap and swimming costume on, and deformed feet as black as coal !

Has the care of the feet anything to do with health ? it may be asked. Yes ! in the first place, feet that have not been hardened give rise to many kinds of chills and worse illnesses, because they soon get cold, and cannot stand being wet, and in the next place, tender feet, suffering from one or more of the defects unfortunately so well known, render an otherwise capable body almost entirely helpless.

The greatest and most important part of what the feet require, however, the daily bath provides. One ought in addition to pay attention to the nails, and remove hard skin after the weekly warm bath or at any rate once a month. Otherwise ingrowing nails, inflammation, etc. will sooner or later make the guilty parties rue their neglect.

Besides which, if you do not give the toes the air and freedom of movement which they, like the rest of the body, require, you will gradually induce perspiring feet, one of the most distressing complaints resulting from dirt, that exist. When you come home in the evening, you ought always to change your shoes and stockings at once, or if summer go about with bare feet, or else simply with sandals (flat leather soles with a few straps)—this is a very cheaply purchased comfort ; the toes will very soon perform gymnastic movements on their own account, while you sit writing or reading. Ugly, angular, hard, or raw toes soon grow round, soft and nice, through the use of stockings with a division for each toe (like gloves).

I am not going to trench further on the question of grown-up people's footwear. They insist, after all, on reserving to themselves the right of wearing shoes too small and too tight, and this applies also to stockings. But I should like to put in a word for the innocent little one. The Chinese often squeeze the feet of their children, to keep them short ; we squeeze them in another direction. It is six of one and half a dozen of the other ! Wherever you go, you see babies lying asleep in their cradles (when once the poor little things have squalled themselves to sleep), with tight stockings and ready-made laced boots on their feet. The least punishment to which their mothers ought to be condemned should be to sleep a night in bed in stockings and laced boots. In the case of 99 per cent. of mothers it is from motives of vanity that their children wear shoes as small and smart as can be procured, and it would certainly be impossible to get any mother to admit that they are too small, even had one an opportunity of drawing the outline of the foot on paper, and proving how much wider it is than the sole of the shoe.

A bad carriage, a clumsy, hesitating walk, distorted feet, and numberless hours of pain are the penalty of wearing, while growing, shoes that are too small.

Eight Hours' Sleep

This is, on an average, the minimum necessary if you do not wish to burn the candle at both ends. But one may very well sleep seven hours in the summer, and nine in the winter. First-rate physical work cannot be performed unless one has slept well the night before, as I have often found from experience, and I doubt whether correspondingly good mental work can, either, unless with the help of nerve-destroying stimulants. Thousands of soldiers have been made nervous wrecks in the Great War because their leaders, without necessity, deprived them of sufficient sleep. As far as the bed itself is concerned, feather-beds should be avoided, and the head should not be too high. One small pillow is sufficient.

Moderation in Smoking

An old English clergyman, who had smoked as a young man, remarked : " On many a minister's tombstone the words ' Died in the Lord ' are engraved, when the inscription ought rather to be ' Smoked himself to death.' "

All the boys one sees with cigarettes in their mouths—and their number is unfortunately legion—are physical, moral, and intellectual suicides.

A pipe or a cigar after lunch and dinner will hardly hurt a grown-up person ; still, one has a fuller use of one's senses, especially those of taste and smell, if one does not smoke. I have frequently experienced this when in times gone by I have left off smoking for several months while training. If you restrict yourself to a few cigars or pipes a day, or half a dozen cigarettes, they will taste all the better.

SPECIAL REMARKS ON THE APPLICATION OF "MY SYSTEM"

Instructions for Exercising Babies and Children

and some very valuable information concerning their upbringing are contained in "My System for Children," which is issued by the publishers of this book, from whom all particulars may be had on application.

For Old People

Fat, like rheumatism and stiffness, can be kept at bay by rational physical exercise every day. Most people think that they are too old for gymnastics as soon as they are over thirty. This is a lamentable error. Physical exercise is *the* only unfailing means whereby one can preserve one's youthful strength, activity and buoyancy, both of body and mind. " Yes, but if you have not gone in for this nonsense since you were a boy, it cannot be any use to set about it when you are fifty and begin to feel old ! " But that is just it—it can !

I have received hundreds of letters from both men and women, of ages ranging from fifty to eighty-five years, declaring that by the use of " My System " they have become as if rejuvenated, and the only complaint they have to make is that they had not become acquainted with the System before they grew so old.

Amongst the pupils at my Institute I remember a lady, a bishop and a colonel who all three started the exercises when about eighty-four years old. One of them was in six weeks freed from constipation of thirty years' standing.

For Literary and Scientific Men and Artists

The minds of such men work according to other laws, and in higher spheres, than those of the uninitiated, and they are consequently inclined to overlook the fact that their bodies are subject to quite ordinary natural laws. If the body is not looked after, it will eventually rebel against the mind and prevent it from attaining its high goal. Most of the great composers and many poets died in their thirties. How many treasures of sound and how many valuable literary productions the world has lost simply because they took no thought for the health of their bodies !

It is especially advantageous for singers to develop their abdominal muscles and their chest.

The *Hygienic Sense* is not one that is acquired in the study. Unfortunately it is only too often lacking in those quarters where it might be of most use, that is to say, among the Sanitary Authorities themselves.

In many countries Physical Culture is a subject of scientific interest, whereas in scientific circles in Denmark it is a *terra incognita*. And yet there is matter in it for no end of theses and treatises, which would have, into the bargain, a chance of proving considerably more generally useful than, for example, " The Eye of the Cod " or " The Vegetation of Madeira."*

For Office Workers

" Surely you do not want to saddle us with still more work ; we sit and toil all day as it is and have barely time to eat !" To this objection I would reply : Listen ! When towards evening you are feeling tired and stiff from stooping, is it not a great relief for a moment (take care though that the chief does not see !) to throw yourself back in your chair and stretch out your arms and legs ? Yet it is a very considerable muscular exertion, you can positively hear your joints crack. The quarter of an hour's extra work, which I have the audacity to try and impose on you, is of a similar nature, and has a similar, but a thousand times greater effect. The town office type is often a sad phenomenon. Prematurely bent, with shoulders and hips awry from his dislocating position on the office stool, pale, with pimply face and pomatumed head, thin neck protruding from a collar that an ordinary man could use as a cuff, and swaggering dress in the latest fashion flapping round the sticks that take the place of arms and legs ! At a more advanced age the spectacle is still more pitiable ; the fashion in dress can be followed no longer, because a family must be fed ; the eyes are dull, and the general appearance is either still more sunken and shrivelled, or else fat, flabby, and pallid, and enveloped in an odour of old paper, putrefied skin-grease, and bad breath. *But things need not be so !*

There is no necessity for work to leave so unpleasant a mark on a man. I was in an office for seventeen years myself. Only spend one poor little fifteen minutes a day in the way I have advised, and life will have much real pleasure to offer you, too !

And then you must try to make your principal understand that if he requires you to sit and inhale bad air all day, from ignorance, or to save the expense of ventilation, it is his fault if you get ill, now that you yourself are doing all you can in your spare time to improve your health !

What applies to people in offices applies likewise to those engaged in literary or other writing work, or in sitting or standing employment indoors.

For those devoted to Athletic Sports

Everyone who is acquainted with the newest and best methods of rowing, swimming, putting the shot, throwing the hammer, the disc, or the 56-lb. weight, knows quite well that the greatest tests of strength in such exercises can only be successfully met by allowing the chief work to fall on the muscles of the legs *and* trunk, whereas the man who, by dint of practising with heavy iron weights, or through Sandow's system, has acquired abnormally thick and knotty arm muscles, ignominiously fails. I have myself been an adept in all these athletics, so can speak from experience.

Perhaps it is not so well known that it is also in the highest degree

*Subjects actually submitted by candidates for the degree of Doctor of Medicine in Denmark.

advantageous for runners, quick walkers, and jumpers to have strong muscles round the waist. By means of the " Corset Exercises " (the name under which I include all the exercises which develop the above-mentioned muscles), a man can keep himself in training throughout the winter, even if he has no opportunity of running in the open air. What generally makes a runner or other devotee of foot-sports, who is not in good training, give up, is not so much want of breath, or tired legs, as those well-known uncomfortable sensations in the abdomen, the diaphragm and the sides and loins, which are summed up in the word " stitch."

In January, 1904, in thick winter clothes and heavy boots, I ran seven miles one hundred and twenty yards over very hilly country through snow and slush, in one hour, and although I had not run for three months, did not feel the least " stitch," simply because I had done my " Corset Exercises " every day. In my younger days, when I was much lighter, but did not do these exercises, I should have got the stitch, under similar circumstances, before I had done a quarter of the distance. I am now (1916) fifty years of age, but still always fit for running or sculling five miles at a fair speed, keeping myself in condition simply by doing " My System " every day.

In selecting the exercises, I have endeavoured to pick out those likely to constitute the best preparation for young people wishing to attain proficiency in the above-mentioned health-giving and recreative physical exercises. Every athlete will find that following up " My System " is the easiest way of keeping himself in condition through the winter, and at the same time of developing the muscles he most stands in need of. In connection herewith, I can show, as curiosities, letters in my possession from many elderly gymnasts and athletes in which the writers inform me that formerly, despite a zealous pursuit of sport, they always had to complain of indigestion or constipation, and that their digestions only became regular after they had practised " My System " for some time.

I must *seriously warn athletes against taking too much exercise* without sufficient rest, food, and sleep ; this is likely to produce a state of affairs (staleness) which makes one fall an easy prey to illness, and is a poor advertisement for any kind of sport, even if one has beaten the record. The question is not so much one of accomplishing, while training, a considerable or protracted and difficult task every day, as of getting the body into such a condition that it is able, without ill effects, to perform the required work when the time comes (for instance, in a race or competition). These principles are often greatly sinned against, and there is much to be learnt in this respect from the Americans, who are the finest athletic sportsmen in the world, and who lay most stress on bringing the *entire* body into a condition of the highest possible degree of health and vitality.

Many sportsmen, also, upset their hearts because they take no care to breathe properly. At the Olympic Games of 1906 it appeared that nearly all the participants, excepting the Americans, suffered from distension, or other defects, of the heart. Those who carry out " My System " according to directions will acquire the good habit of inhaling and exhaling deeply, both *during* the exercises as well as *immediately after* them. The reason why I have been able to take part, for a whole generation, in many and various hard and often protracted contests

c

without inflicting the slightest injury upon my heart, is because I have always from childhood paid strict attention to correct respiration.

For Women to Remember

If only half the time that is now spent in dressing, or in curling and other ruination of the hair, was devoted to a sensible care of the body, there would be fewer unhappy marriages and fewer unsatisfactory children. This Vale of Tears would become a Paradise. All women wish for beauty, harmonious proportions, and a good figure, but possibly not one in a hundred of them knows what these really consist of, and that the only means of acquiring them—and in the case of older women, keeping them—is a daily bath, rubbing the skin, and all-round bodily exercise, together with fresh air and sunshine.

The present generation of grown-up women is doubtless almost past praying for. But perhaps, ladies, for your daughters' sakes, it may interest you to know that in twenty years' time men will have advanced so far in knowledge and appreciation of Hygiene, that they will no longer rest content with compassionating the woman who has made havoc of herself by wearing a corset (even if she have not tight-laced) and high heels, but they will dub it stupidity, slovenliness, and idleness on her part to go about in a corset and neglect her daily bath and exercise. It will be an exceedingly uncomfortable position for a newly married woman to find herself in if her husband has to point out to her how low she stands in the scale of civilisation, as regards the care of her health and beauty, and, baldly stated, her cleanliness, beneath her outward finery. A woman who leaves off her corset is, however, in ill case if she does not get something else in its stead to keep her warm and hold her body upright and together. Warmth comes quickly enough when the skin is awakened out of its lethargy by the bath and rubbing exercises. Medical books state that muscles which will support the body gradually develop of themselves, if the corset be left off, but these muscles, it is true, make their appearance very slowly or not at all, unless one performs exercises, such as those I have indicated, which are specially calculated to produce them, and with the help of which one can acquire a "muscular corset" in a few months. The secret of the beautiful figures of the female statues of antiquity lies in the fact that they all possess a corset of this kind in lieu of the modern expensive, ugly, perishable, uncomfortable, and unhealthy substitute.

"But we really have not time!"

Yes! you have! The more you have to do, the better you will understand how to arrange your time so that there will be one quarter of an hour to spare. And when you have once properly begun you will look forward eagerly every day to this quarter of an hour and especially to the extraordinary agreeable sensation that the rubbing produced all over the body.

It stands to reason that women, at certain times, should omit the full bath and the exercises demanding most exertion, and should content themselves with the easiest of the rubbing exercises.

This plea of lack of time very seldom indeed holds good, when you come to enquire more closely into matters. Many mothers declare that they have no time to bathe themselves and their children every day, to do exercise with them, brush their teeth, see that their bowels work properly, get them out in the fresh air in all weathers, etc., but the same mothers have plenty of time to devour one novel after another, to chat with others of the same way of thinking on the stairs or at the corners of the streets, to parade the town, or go to tea-shops.

For Cyclists

The bicycle is a splendid means for getting from the town atmosphere out into the fresh country air, quickly and independently of trains, and for returning again when duty calls. And as a means of conveyance for tourists it is invaluable. In other respects, however, its importance for the health is not very great. I rode a high bicycle as early as 1883, and afterwards, for many years, a safety both in winter and summer. But it dawned upon me by degrees that as a daily means of getting about, the cycle tricked me out of the good exercise that a quick walk to and from business provides.

Rational games and sports on foot give a classical contour to the legs. A brisk walk—not to speak of really quick walking—in addition to those of the legs, brings many of the other muscles of the body into play, whereas cycling overdevelops some few of the leg muscles, the other parts of the body being fatigued and prejudiced by being kept either constantly on the strain or wholly inoperative. A man who gets no exercise but cycling cannot avoid sundry parts of his body being defective, and he may fall a victim to divers illnesses. It is therefore still more important for the cyclist than for the pedestrian to exercise the muscles round the body, and those of the chest, the back, and the shoulders, every day. I do not believe this can be procured in any easier or more effective manner than by following out " My System."

For Country People

Dear dwellers in the country ! You are world-renowned for your skill in cultivating the soil, breeding cattle, and making butter.* You have also the reputation of being shrewd and sensible, and of not caring to spend money on useless things.

Then why will you swallow all the expensive medicine that the doctor often only recommends you because you would otherwise say that he does not know his business ? Hear what some of the shrewdest doctors in the world have said. *Sir Morell Mackenzie* (the Emperor Frederick's doctor) said : " If there were not a single drop of medicine in the world, the death-rate would be lower !" and *Dr. Titus* (the Court Physician at Dresden) said : " Three-quarters of the human race are killed by medicine." Nearly all patent medicine is poison ; the more one takes, the less it helps in the place required, while the whole of the rest of the body gets poisoned.

It is scandalous that there should be so much illness in the country, where every condition exists for leading a perfectly healthy life. *The principal reason is that you really have not the least notion of caring for your skin.*

It is bad enough that you have such a horror of fresh air in your rooms, but this is counteracted in a great measure by the air being so much better than in the town, the moment that you poke your nose

---

* This remark applies of course more particularly to the Danes, who, as is well known, are very skilful farmers. £7,600,000 worth of butter, for instance, is exported every year.

outside the door. And you nearly all get enough exercise, even if it be only partial. Among the factory workers and the poor in large towns illness can be excused, but not among you. You get poisoned and out of sorts because you neglect your skin. And instead of seeking health by washing, grooming, and hardening it every day (which you do for your horses and cattle, and in places even for your pigs), you gorge yourselves with still more poison in the shape of medicine, and muffle yourselves up in still more unnecessary clothing. The result, of course, is that illness will seize hold of you still more readily next time. One of your greatest inflictions, so much discussed and written about just now, I mean Consumption, owes to this its extraordinary dissemination in the country. *Dr. Dettweiler*, the celebrated tuberculosis specialist, said : " The tuberculosis patient is as much skin-sick as lung sick." Neglect of the skin destroys a man's power of resisting bacilli.

Dr. P. Niemeyer says : " Dread of fresh air is the chief cause of tuberculosis. He who combats this dread does as much for the prevention of the disease as he who fights the bacilli."

What hotbeds of disease the small, overcrowded, and practically unventilated village schoolrooms are ! The air is either supersaturated with the varied emanations arising from crowds of dirty children, often mingled with steam from wet clothes, and greased boots, or else it is heavy with smoke and dust from the stove. If a sensible schoolmaster attempts to open the windows during a lesson, he gets all the parents down upon him.

The gymnastics pursued in many places with such ardour *might* be of benefit to the health of you country people ; but as things are, they tend to do more harm than good, by reason of your very deficient comprehension of the care of your skin and the need for fresh air. I have frequently witnessed voluntary gymnastic exercises of the sort in the country. Those participating in them would be inhaling vigorously the air of the little room, full of dust and laden with noxious emanations and tobacco-smoke. The perspiration would pour off them, but not one of them would take a bath afterwards. They would put on their clothes again, and allow the perspiration to dry on them and deposit still another cake of poisonous matter on the body, on the top of all the old layers from previous lessons. When I remarked to the most active of the gymnasts that I wondered at the constitutions they must have, not all to fall mortally ill together, he admitted that he certainly very often did feel unwell afterwards.

For Travellers

I have often heard commercial travellers and others, whose occupation obliges them to be away from home for long together, complain that they had simply no opportunity of strengthening their bodies by gymnastics or sports, and that they often came to provincial towns where it was difficult and entailed waste of time to get a bath, which, as everyone knows, one stands in special need of after a railway journey. Here I believe that " My System " will supply a want. There is no apparatus to be carried about or set up. As soon as you come from the railway station into your room at the hotel, you undress, stand on a carpet, and slap the body all over with a wet towel—or you can without any inconvenience carry a small india rubber bath with you—dry yourself, and go through the rubbing exercises. As you are dressing again afterwards, you can wash your face, neck, hands, and feet with soap in the wash-hand basin. As you see, the fatigues of the journey take the place of the exercises before the bath, but if you are staying several days in the same place you will of course go through the whole System either morning or evening.

For Fat and Thin People

How can the same cause have two directly opposite effects ? Don't you know the fable of the Indian who was so astonished to see the European blow warm and cold with the same mouth, first when his fingers were cold and then when the soup was too hot ?

I divide people, as far as their habit of body is concerned, into the following main classes : (1) The plump, (2) the thin, (3) the muscularly fat, (4) the skinny, and (5) the flabbily fat. There are, of course, many intermediate stages ; for instance, one sees people who actually in the upper part of their bodies belong to the one class, and in the lower to another. The bodies of those belonging to the first class have full, long muscles, which are quite soft when in repose, the muscles of the second class are short, well marked, and often overtrained. The third class have a layer of fat above and between otherwise really good muscles, whereas the two worst classes have practically no muscles at all. It is often very difficult to classify correctly anyone wearing clothes. Thus a great many men commonly come under the description of " strong " who, from a physical point of view, are no good whatever, while apparently lean men may be athletes. One and the same individual can change classes from many different causes, i.e. : if a man in Class 1 be not careful, and does not lead a healthy life, he either goes over into Class 3 or (according to his age) too soon into Class 2. Class 4, with good living, becomes Class 5, and this last again, through illness or starvation. Class 4. The models of the antique statues, both men and women, belonged to Class 1 ; of the models of the present day, the men are generally Class 2, and the women Class 5. With sensible training (following out my directions, for instance), people of all Classes can be transformed to Class 1 (with the exception in certain cases of those in Class 2). People in Class 4 will develop the muscles of their bodies and limbs, and thus grow stouter and heavier.

As far as fat people are concerned, they must first ascertain to which class they belong, as people of the fifth Class must always proceed very gradually and cautiously.

People of the third Class can generally bear to get rid of fat *quickly* by long runs, sweat-baths, and rigid training. But the troublesome part of this violent method is that the fat round the waist is the last to budge, whilst it is just that that one wishes to get rid of *first*. So that this training, too, should be supplemented by my " Corset and rubbing exercises."

The most striking proofs with which I have hitherto become acquainted that " My System " will reduce superfluous fat are the following :—

Signor Contini, Director of the Maison Alexandre in Rome, who in two years, solely by the daily practice of " My System," reduced his weight from 123 kilograms (270 lbs.) to 78 kilograms (171 lbs.)—a loss of 99 lbs.

And a captain of the Royal Engineers, India, who reduced his weight in eighteen months from twenty-two stone to twelve stone, losing no less than 140 lbs. I could scarcely believe him until he showed me an old photo.

Both of them at the same time found that their capacity for work and their vitality had immensely increased. Besides which, it may be seen any day how people gain two to two-and-a-half inches in chest circumference while at the same time losing just as much in waist measurements.

Whereas it is a good thing for fat people to lose fat, it is a bad thing for these people to gain fat. It is true that they ought to gain weight in order to become normal, but what they put on should be sound flesh, consisting of muscular fibres and tissues and not fatty substance. They are two quite different things just as diametrically opposite each other as " Health " and " Illness." Let us therefore for Heaven's sake discriminate between " fat " and " flesh."

I will now first give a little synopsis of the various ways to get rid of the harmful, or at all events superfluous fat, and afterwards I will give a few hints how to become normal, by putting on the right sort of flesh.

Accumulation of fat is due to want of the right method of exercise. Even healthy persons with excellent organs of assimilation will grow fat, notwithstanding the fact that they do not over-indulge in eating or drinking.

Now fat can be removed by :—

(1) Dieting (seldom very effectual, never pleasing ; may affect the temper badly).
(2) Protracted Fasting (very effectual ; but is dangerous if not done under proper scientific control).
(3) Turkish and other perspiration baths (not very effectual unless combined with other methods ; affect heart if not strong ; may cause colds).
(4) Fat-reducing drugs (check the work of the intestines so that much can be eaten without being assimilated ; are poisonous and ruin the digestive organs in the long run).
(5) Proper Exercise.

Long walks are not of much use for reducing the fat of the upper body. Such exercises increase the appetite so that more food is put into the stomach, but it strengthens the legs and improves the health generally, so do not miss the walk, besides doing the right exercises to get rid of the fat.

The fat disappears by :—

(1) Working the muscles which are situated directly below the layers of fat ;
(2) Hard self-massage to loosen and bring into circulation the fatty tissues, and
(3) Deep exhalations to get rid of the waste stuff burnt up in the lungs.

After practice, these three things can be done simultaneously to save time, as in my Rubbing Exercises. Sweaters are not necessary. The evaporations will leave through the naked skin, even if you do not observe any drops. Further, these proper fat-reducing exercises strengthen the general health and increase the vitality.

Now, the means to get an ideal, the true normal figure, one of First Class, the happy medium of bodily form, neither too thin nor fat, is again proper exercise, which of course must be supported by proper food and rest. There is no fear that the food will not be assimilated, because the very same exercises will stimulate all the organs of digestion and metabolism, and the other functions, especially sleep, will be perfect too, if only you will allow the necessary time, because the very same exercises teach you to relax the body and limbs completely, and they purify the blood of the poisons which otherwise rack the nerves.

It is the big muscles of the trunk, the shoulders, chest, abdomen, flanks, back, hips and loins, which if properly developed, create the beautiful harmonious figures of the classical statues, both male and female. And next in importance are the muscle groups of the limbs, situated nearest the trunk. Exercising these muscles will make the upper arms and thighs full and plump, but the limbs will be gradually slender towards the hands and feet—again the true classical shape.

The form of a muscle in repose is always harmonious, whereas the fat settles without symmetry in ugly bulks. This fact is always forgotten, especially by the ladies who want to get plump. They imagine that " muscle " must be something male, hard and knotty. But what an unhappy mistake ! It is just big muscles in a state of repose that makes the divine form of any Venus.

The whole of the matter is that too much exercise, and wrong exercises, will have bad effects. The average should be ten to twenty minutes' home gymnastics and half to one hour of open-air walking daily, supplemented by some week-end game or hobby. But do not tire the muscles or make them " dry " and hard by working them for hours without rest.

General Remarks on the Application of " My System "

It will be explained later on, in the description of the separate exercises, how beginners and more advanced workers, of different degrees of strength and according to age, should undertake them. Attention is drawn to the advice given to beginners on page 52. If sufficient attention be paid to these matters, the System will be found suited to practically all, irrespective of age or sex. People suffering from acute illness, or from such grave organic defects as heart disease, cavities in the lungs, or ulceration of the bowels, must, of course, be excepted, and should in any case ask their doctor's advice.

SPECIAL EXERCISES FOR SPECIAL COMPLAINTS

To cure a chronic ailment permanently, we must know the causes and then remove them, and thus eradicate the ailment and prevent it from developing again.

Now, one of the most common superstitions is, that to each different ailment correspond one or two special exercises, by the practice of which such ailment may be cured. I think the idea originates from the old belief that an ailment is something which suddenly falls upon an innocent individual, and to make it disappear again one only has to open the right drawer, find the right box and swallow the right pill or drug, which has been prepared especially for the ailment in question. People are often really offended when I tell them that it is not a special exercise for the limb, or part of the body where the pain is felt, that they need, but a general toning up of all the vital and eliminating organs.

There are, of course, special cases of muscular weakness or bodily deformities where certain exercises have a very good effect, whereas others are better left alone, but even then general exercises for strengthening the heart and lungs, improving the digestion and increasing the circulation, are of the first importance; otherwise the muscles and tissues at the weak spot will get no proper nourishment, but only become sore and strained by overdoing the " special " exercise, and eventually they will atrophy instead of growing stronger.

However, all the common chronic complaints which arise from auto-intoxication ("self-poisoning" of the blood, and thereby the whole body, from the digestive channel, bad teeth and gums, old toxins or other sources) are simply cured and prevented by purifying the whole system. Rheumatic, uric acid or gouty pains may have very various names and be felt in different parts of the body and limbs, because the circulating poisons will always find the weak, or accidentally damaged, spot and make an attack there.

Hence the best " special " exercises for arthritis, lumbago, neuralgia, neuritis, sciatica, rheumatic gout and all other similar complaints, most diseases of the kidneys and many forms of boils, eczema, rash, palpitation of the heart, spots before the eyes and noises in the head, dropsy in the legs, etc., are deep breathing and skin-rubbing exercises, combined with bendings and twistings of the trunk, because such exercises enormously increase the activities of the three channels through which waste matters and poisons are got rid of, viz., the skin, lungs and bowels, and simultaneously the fourth of the eliminating organs, the kidneys, are relieved of the poisons with which they used to be overloaded.

In the same way these trunk exercises (Nos. 1, 3, 4, 6, 7, 11, 12, 13, 16, 17 and 18) and knee-bendings, all with deep breathing, are really the best " specials " for remedying all the chronic ailments caused by bad circulation and faulty metabolism—such as anæmia, chilblains, diabetes, biliousness and most liver complaints. Furthermore, for the most common forms of indigestion (acidity, flatulence, heartburn, dyspepsia, nausea), gastritis, colitis, constipation, and dropped and dilated stomach, these trunk-bendings and twistings, combined with abdominal self-massage and deep-breathing, are the only "special" exercises.

The reason why the correct way of breathing during exercise is so important for the functions of the stomach, liver, intestines and bowels, is, that all these organs are moved and massaged inside, and thus toned up if the lower ribs are completely contracted and in turn fully expanded, and the diaphragm thus forced up and downwards to the utmost limits.

Sometimes the above-mentioned ailments develop if a nerve is mechanically affected by some fault in the framework of the body—whether from birth or caused by an accident. In such cases an osteopath should readjust the structure of the bones, as otherwise the full benefit will not be derived from the exercises.

Again, deep breathings combined with skin-rubbing exercises are the best "special" exercises to harden oneself against catarrh and prevent all diseases which may follow a cold, in that the power of resistance against change of temperature, and the germ-killing ability of the blood, is highly increased.

If the bacilli get the upper hand because the person is weak or has for the moment weakened himself by overwork, too little sleep, too much alcohol, or other sins against Hygiene, and an acute illness follows, perhaps with fever, then the best thing is to go to bed immediately and send for the doctor. Under these circumstances, even if the patient is in the habit of doing my exercises daily, he must drop them for a little while. The advantage of having done them regularly lies then in the fact that all the body processes are so lively and the vital organs so active that the patient will recover in a few days' time, whereas it would take other people weeks or months.

Finally, let me once more emphasize that there are no single special exercises for single special ailments. Only in a very few cases are some exercises more effectual than others.

My exercises are so selected that the whole series is really "special exercises" for every common chronic ailment or disability, because they make the whole body healthy, strong and perfect by improving all the vital processes, by strengthening every muscle and bone, and by toning up every organ. Then any ailment, weakness or deformity will gradually disappear of itself. To make an individual healthy is to cure his ill, and in making the body perfect, fat people will become slender, thin people will become muscular and plump, those who stoop will become erect, and so on.

LIST OF CHRONIC AILMENTS AND BODILY DEFECTS AND INFIRMITIES SUCCESSFULLY TREATED WITH MULLER EXERCISES

Under the control of the patient's own Doctor or upon the advice of a Specialist

Now please remember that I am no doctor of medicine, and that I do not pose as such. When, therefore, in the following pages I give a few practical hints to sufferers from some of the most common of these chronic ailments and bodily defects, do not forget that my experience concerns mainly exercise and breathing. Therefore, if you will use this book for curing yourself, you should get the advice of your own doctor or a specialist about the best diet, what medicine or tonic to take (if any), how to bathe, etc., etc.

ABDOMEN, distended. The best exercises are No. 3, No. 6, with both legs at once, No. 12 and No. 18, when done very quickly. See the test described under Exercise No. 12.

ACIDITY. (See Indigestion).

ACNE.

ADENOIDS, beginning. Study "My Breathing System.'

ADHESIONS.

ANÆMIA. Young persons, mostly girls, suffering from this must gradually perform all the eighteen exercises (but only the milder degrees of the first eight) in order to improve the assimilation of food and increase the metabolism and general circulation, without tiring themselves out. Long hours in the open air, with deep breathing without strenuous exercise, and in the summer, sunbathing, not dressed, but naked (see "MY SUNBATHING AND FRESH AIR SYSTEM"), are beneficial.

ANKLES, weak. The special foot exercises explained on page 114 are excellent. But all the vital organs should first be toned up, and the circulation, and the blood itself improved by some months' performance of the regular eighteen exercises of the "System." Otherwise the tissues of the weak spot will not get sufficient nourishment to make up for the extra strain, and the lamentable result will be increased feebleness.

APPENDICITIS, beginning.

ARTHRITIS. See the foregoing chapter.

ARTERIO-SCLEROSIS.

ASSIMILATION, bad.

ASTHMA, nervous. Real asthma in old people with the air pipe damaged can be healed no more than lungs with cavities. But the sporadic attacks of asthma, very often due to poisoning of the nerves that control the muscles of expiration, can be cured by purifying the whole body (see "Auto-intoxication").

In the case of young people, the cause is often simply lack of control or development of the breathing muscles. It is then sufficient to learn how to exhale completely, and the attacks will not occur again.

It is recommended to study "My Breathing System."

ATROPHY.

AUTO-INTOXICATION. The human body can be "self-poisoned" in various ways.

There is a certain amount of poison in most of what we eat and drink, and, if the waste matters are not quickly eliminated, they will soon become "poisonous." The poisons will pass into the blood, be circulated through the body, affect the heart and irritate the nerves, and attack any weak part of the body. All feelings of tiredness, both local and general, giddiness, brain-fag, many headaches and "rheumatic" pains, much insomnia and depression are due to such poisons. The best way to get rid of them is to ensure perfect action of the main eliminating organs, viz. : lungs, skin, bowels and kidneys, and to effect this, all the eighteen exercises are necessary. "Auto-intoxication" follows in the wake of all the various digestive troubles, sluggish liver, wrongly-acting gall bladder and bad teeth, but worry, anger, fear and sorrow, are also liable to produce chemical poisons inside the human body.

BACKACHE.

BILIOUSNESS. See the foregoing chapter.

BLOOD PRESSURE, faulty.

BLUSHING.

BOILS, if not caused by poisons from outside. See the foregoing chapter.

BOW LEGS. When the digestion, assimilation, metabolism and circulation are perfected and the blood purified by performing the eighteen exercises for some time, the following special exercises can be performed :

Stand upright with hands on hips, and feet as much apart as possible, toes pointing outwards. Now drag the feet close together by little shuffling movements of each foot alternately, each movement being only a few inches in length. The soles of the feet while being dragged should be pressed hard against the floor, keeping the knees rigid the whole time. Then stand astride again and repeat the exercise several times, until tired.

Here is another excellent exercise for strengthening and straightening the legs. Lie down on the floor, having the assistance of a friend. The legs are opened as far as possible, sideways, and again closed under mutual and powerful resistance. *You should have the feet outside.* Repeat it until tired. Do not forget to breathe steadily and fully. If you have no friend to give you assistance, you can perform the second half of the third degree of exercise No. 6 (with the legs pressed together in the downward movement) an extra number of times, say fifty times each day with pauses of rest, of course, but pressing as hard as possible and trying to get the knees together. You ought to have special heels made for your boots, the heels being higher on the outside than the inner. When lying in bed on the back and sleeping, you may have a broad elastic band round your knees, so that there is a constant pressure inwards.

Swimming and dancing is good for bow legs; but riding and football should be avoided.

BRAIN FAG. See "Auto-intoxication."

BREATH, short. Study "My Breathing System" and perform the exercises explained therein.

BRONCHITIS (chronic). Study "My Breathing System" and perform the exercises explained therein.

CARRIAGE, bad. Exercise No. 8 should be omitted, whereas Exercises Nos. 1, 2, 5, 7, 11, 13, 15, 16, 17 and 18 and the special Neck exercises (see page 111), are excellent, if performed correctly. Do not sit in a too stiff and erect position when resting, as this will only tire your weak back-muscles.

CATARRH (in nose, bronchi, stomach, intestines). See the foregoing chapter.

CHEST, weak, narrow, pigeon and other deformities. Study "My Breathing System" and perform the exercises explained therein.

CHILBLAINS. See the foregoing chapter.

CIRCULATION, bad. See the foregoing chapter.

COLDS, liability to. See the foregoing chapter.

COLITIS. See the foregoing chapter.

CONGESTION, in head, throat, etc. Downward bending, as in Exercise No. 11, should be omitted during the first weeks and replaced by the special foot exercises (see page 114). Exercise No. 9, and the squatting of No. 10, are very good. The worst fault is holding the breath.

CONSTIPATION. This may be due to one or more of five various causes. (1) Lack of proper exercise for the abdomen. Exercises Nos. 3, 4. 6, 11 and 18 are the most effective in this case. (2) Too much one-sided exercise with free perspiration. For instance, long-distance runners or walkers are sometimes constipated, because the fæces become too hard and dry. (3) A wrong diet, i.e., too refined food, of which the greater part is absorbed so that finally there is nothing on which the bowels can act. In such cases more bulky or volumi-nous food should be taken (vegetables, porridge, brown or black bread). You must be careful not to fall in the Scylla of indigestion, in evading the Charybdis of constipation. (4) The habit so common amongst thin persons, or soldiers, of keeping the abdomen con-stantly indrawn and rigid, so that the intestines and bowels are kept immovable and without proper room for working. The pupil must first of all learn to relax the abdominal wall and to move the lower ribs, and thereby the diaphragm, to the utmost limits when breath-ing during exercise. (5) The right time is simply missed (for going to the stool), a common cause amongst women and children. The bowels should be educated to act once (or twice) a day exactly at the same time, and when Nature calls, she should be obeyed immediately. It if is held over for only a few minutes, constipation may already be established.

CONSUMPTION, beginning. Study "My Breathing System" and per-form the exercises explained therein.

CRAMPS.

CRETINISM.

CURVATURE of spine. The best exercises for straightening the spine are Nos. 1, 4, 7, 11, 12, 13, 16 and 17. A good special exercise is to hang by the hands in the Roman Rings or a Trapeze, with arms stretched and all muscles of the shoulders, trunk and legs relaxed. The feet may rest on the floor, but the whole weight of the body should pull downwards from the arms. Then swing the body to and fro, or round in circles. A slight curvature is very common amongst school children who seldom give themselves time to take up a proper sitting position with the legs square in front of the body, but allow both legs to remain on one side, with the opposite shoulder and elbow thrust out to the other side, so that the body is kept for long periods in a twisted position, especially when writing. In severe cases one side of the chest is underdeveloped. Then Exercise No. 4, 1st or 2nd degree " B," should be used as a special exercise, but without change in the breathing, so that expiration always takes place when bending to the side least developed, and inspiration each time the trunk is bent to the other side.

DEPRESSION, general. See "Auto-intoxication."

DIABETES. Doctors' prescriptions on diet are very important here. All my exercises which move the trunk in the waistline, thereby toning up the internal organs of assimilation and metabolism, are good for this condition. Further, deep breathing and skin-rubbing exercises, air and sun-baths help very materially.

DIARRHŒA, tendency to.

DYSPEPSIA. (See Indigestion.)

EMPHYSEMA. Study "My Breathing System" and perform the exercises explained therein.

EPILEPSY.

ECZEMA. When Eczema is caused by self-poisons, it can be cured by exercise (see the foregoing chapter). Eczema caught by contagion must have the doctor's special treatment

FLATFOOTEDNESS. Many people erroneously imagine that they—or their children—have flat feet. The short but highly arched foot is by no means the classical shape. The ancient Greek statues, both male and female, have always long feet, with a rather low instep. Now, to ascertain if your feet are really " flat," make the following test : Dip the whole of the soles into water and walk a few steps with your natural gait. If the humid prints on the floor are widest in the middle, then you are flat-footed, but if they are narrow in the middle, you are certainly not. The best exercise to cure this defect is the special foot exercise (see page 114). Or simply stand with heels together, rise high upon the toes while you inhale, lower the heels again slowly, exhaling, and repeat up to fifty times. As to the necessary preliminary exercises, see "Ankles, weak."

FLATULENCE. (See Indigestion.)

GASTRITIS (internal stasis). See the foregoing chapter.

GIDDINESS. (See "Auto-intoxication.")

GOITRE.

GOUT. See the foregoing chapter.

HAY FEVER.

HEADACHE. (See "Auto-intoxication.")

HEART, weak, fat, distended, displaced, nervous. Study "My Breathing System" and perform the exercises explained therein.

HEARTBURN. (See Indigestion.)

HAEMORRHOIDS. These are, more often than not, due to bad circulation and to undue strain in trying to get an action of the bowels. In bad cases the surgeon's knife is the best remedy, but milder attacks can be remedied and prevented by improving the circulation and curing the constipation. (See notes on these items.)

HERNIA. In young people this may be cured by gradually strengthening the abdominal wall by Exercises Nos. 1, 3, 6, 7, and 11 (but keep for a long time to the easy degree of Nos. 3 and 6). All jerky movements, holding of the breath, severe coughing and lifting of heavy things should be avoided. Middle-aged and elderly people, even with double hernia, can derive general benefit to their health by doing the whole " System," but they must wear their truss while exercising.

IMBECILITY.

INDIGESTION. Nowhere is a vicious circle so easily established as in this large group of complaints. A sufferer from any " stomach " trouble will soon get bad-tempered, and this will immediately have a slackening influence on all the physical processes, and first of all upon the digestion. Some cases are started by worrying, but most cases are due to eating too much, too quickly or too often, or eating food not suitable to the individual. The afternoon tea meal causes indigestion in thousands of middle-aged people. Three, or even two meals a day are sufficient for the average grown-up brain worker, or idle individual. By all means drink the tea, and have a smoke, but do not eat. One biscuit alone will stir the whole machinery and disturb the sorely needed rest of the stomach. The feeling of hunger is often only a false one, due to fermentation of food previously eaten. It will gradually disappear even if you do not eat very soon.

Most cases can be cured either by dieting and fasting, or by the right exercises (see the foregoing chapter). By the last method, the whole body will simultaneously be strengthened, and when, after some months' time, the digestive organs are toned up, the person can, with moderation, eat and drink just what he likes best. Long walks or protracted games are not always able to cure indigestion. The appetite will be increased, so that still more is put into the poor stomach. I have had several pupils who walked from three to eight miles a day and always suffered from indigestion, but a few minutes' performance daily of my trunk exercises very soon cured them.

INSOMNIA. Only cases due to auto-intoxication can be directly cured by exercises. If the cause is mental, it must first be removed, otherwise exercising, if not very gentle, may aggravate the complaint. The six weeks' programme (see page 52) should be spread over three months.

KIDNEYS (loose, weak, gravel in). See the foregoing chapter.

KNOCK-KNEES. Preliminary exercising the same as for " Bow Legs." The best exercises of " My System " are No. 6, third degree, trying to press the feet together each time the legs meet, with the addition of the squatting of No. 10, and Nos. 14 and 15, with powerful stroking of the legs. The following is a good special exercise : The Deep Knee-bending (explained on page 60), with the thighs forced well apart. Further, I should recommend the sufferer to wear boots with the heels made higher on the inner side than outer. When lying upon the back, sleeping, have the ankles tied together, or kept together by a broad elastic band, and place a firm pillow between the knees. Riding on horseback is a splendid exercise, but cycling is not, and rowing or sculling with a sliding seat is also very good. The knees should be well opened when the body is brought forwards. Swimming is highly recommended, because it tends to straighten the legs, whatever the deformity. And if the legs are not weak, football will be also very beneficial.

LARYNGITIS (chronic).

LIVER (sluggish, enlarged, congested). See the foregoing chapter.

LUMBAGO. Only the most acute attacks should force you to go to bed. Milder attacks and chronic pains will gradually yield to exercise (see the foregoing chapter). It is not dangerous to do strong bending, twisting and stretching movements, and thus brave the pains, if only you are warm and start gently. If cold, you must avoid jerks and sudden movements. Digging, or any exercise where you remain for long in a bent position, is risky. If perspiring, be careful to finish with a hot bath and change the clothes.

MOUTH-BREATHING. Study " My Breathing System " and practise the exercises explained therein.

MUSCLE-BOUNDNESS. See the chapters on " Relaxation."

NAUSEA. (See " Indigestion.")

NEURALGIA. See the foregoing chapter.

NEURASTHENIA. The six weeks' programme, as explained on page 52, should be spread over six months. If possible, do the exercises between two main meals, not before breakfast. When walking in the open air, practise the deep-breathing very carefully, but sit down every now and then and rest. The most important thing is to get good sleep, which is the only *real* Nerve Tonic in existence. For your own sake, fight shy of patent medicine like poison.

NEURITIS. See the foregoing chapter.

NOISES, in head, ears. See the foregoing chapter.

OBESITY. See chapter " For Fat and Thin People."

OBSTRUCTIONS, in nose. Study " My Breathing System," and let a surgeon examine the nose.

PALPITATION OF HEART. Study " My Breathing System," and see the foregoing chapter.

PERSPIRING, hands and feet. A sufferer from auto-intoxication will get rid of much poisonous matter by perspiring. But if the skin of the whole body is not working properly, the perspiration will seek the channels of least resistance, *i.e.*, where the pores are most numerous, namely in the palms, the soles of the feet, and the armpits. Owing to the concentration of the poisons, the fluid will smell very badly. It is obvious, then, that the cause of the evil will not be removed by treating only the hands and feet. The whole surface of the skin must be toned up, and all the pores opened by daily baths (to be taken hot at first) and skin-rubbing exercises. But first of all the sources of the " auto-intoxication " must be stopped. (See this item, and the foregoing chapter.)

PILES. (See Hæmorrhoids.)

PIMPLES.

PSORIASIS.

RASH. See the foregoing chapter.

RHEUMATISM. (See "Auto-intoxication" and foregoing chapter.

RUPTURE. (See "Hernia.")

SALT CELLARS. When assimilation of the food and circulation of the blood have been improved, the best exercises are Nos. 5, 8 and 13 ; the hard rubbing (pressing) in all rubbing exercises ; and the special neck exercises. Swimming on the back, and the arm movements in Trudgeon-and-Crawl-Swimming are very good.

SCIATICA. See the remarks on Lumbago and the foregoing chapter. The worst thing to do is to sit on a hard seat, or to expose the legs to cold and dampness. But hot baths are beneficial.

SEASICKNESS. Experience shows that those who regularly perform the whole " System," with correct breathing, soon grow immune. Some believe it is because the solar plexus region is so much strengthened. When the ship is rolling, place yourself where the air is fresh, and take deep respirations, inhaling when you rise with a wave, exhaling when you go downwards.

SELF-CONFIDENCE, loss of.

SEXUAL WEAKNESS.

SHOULDER-BLADES, protruding. The cause in children and young people is usually a lack of sufficient muscle flesh to cover these bones. The best exercises are Nos. 5, 10, and 13, and powerful pressing against the body in all the rubbing exercises. Exercise No. 8 should be omitted until the defect has been corrected.

SLEEPLESSNESS. (See " Insomnia.")

SPASMS OF THE PYLORUS.

SPOTS BEFORE THE EYES. See the foregoing chapter.

STATURE, small. I always buy the various " secret " exercises which time after time are advertised by people who " guarantee " to increase the height of anybody. I have never found any exercises better than my Nos. 1, 4, 7, 11, 13, 16, 17 and 18, for this purpose. Most grown-up, elderly and old people increase about an inch during the first months of doing my exercises. Then the limit is reached and no other set of exercises ever invented could add another quarter of an inch. Those under twenty-five years of age can increase by three or even more inches, (1) if they have not yet reached the height of their brothers or sisters, parents or grand-parents ; (2) if they have never before done exercises furthering the growth ; and (3), if besides exercising correctly, they get plenty of good food (properly assimilated) and rest (at least 9 hours' sleep).

STAMMERING, nervous. Study " My Breathing System."

STOMACH, displaced, dilated. See the foregoing chapter.

STOOPING. A very good special exercise is the following : Stand with the heels together and at a distance of about ten inches from a wall (after practice, stand further away). Raise the stretched arms up sideways so that the little fingers slide up along the wall until level with the shoulders, at the same time inhaling fully. Then lower

the arms slowly again while exhaling deeply. Repeat several
times. Later you may rise up on the toes during each inhalation,
and again lower the heels during the exhalations. For further
information, see under "Carriage, bad." Of the neck exercises,
the upward and backward movement of No. 1 is the most effective.

SYNOVITIS.

TENNIS ARM. Rest the bad arm as much as possible, but perform carefully the exercises for improving the general circulation (see the
foregoing chapter), not forgetting the deep knee-bendings. In the
rubbing exercises the stroking and massage should be done with
the sound arm only. And No. 8 can be done as recommended to
one-armed people. But the exercises where the bad arm is moved
without being bent, could be done in full (Exercises Nos. 4, 5 and
7). If the right arm is affected, learn to play with the left, or go
in for some boxing.

THINNESS. See the chapter " For Fat and Thin People."

THROAT, sore.

TUBERCULOSIS, in the lungs. If the disease is not further advanced
than the First Stage, it can be cured by following the advice given
in " My Breathing System."

URIC ACIDS. See the foregoing chapter.

WILL-POWER, lack of.

VARICOSE VEINS, beginning. The majority of cases are caused by
elastic garters. The ordinary ' suspenders " used by men to keep
their socks nice and tight are so especially harmful that most of
those who have worn them for a few months only, will already shew
signs of swelling, owing to the steady pressure upon the main vein.
The man who invented this diabolic appliance has deprived
millions of legs of their fitness and usefulness. The circulation of
the feet will, of course, suffer too, and any wound below the garter
will take a long time in healing. I have got hundreds of pupils
to dispose of them, or at all events to use them only when walking
in the streets, but never when sitting in the office or at home, or
when exercising. I always recommend boys with long woollen
stockings to slip the garters down round the ankles when they are
not running about.

Very bad and painful cases should be operated upon. Elastic
stockings and broad bandages protect and support the legs, but
will not cure. Only mild cases can be cured. The best exercise is
No. 15 with powerful massage upwards. Movement is always good
if not overdone, but standing still with the body's weight upon the
legs should be avoided. When sitting, the feet should, if possible
be placed high up, after the American fashion.

VARICOCELE, beginning.

WATER IN THE LEGS. See foregoing chapter.

WINDSUCKING. Study "My Breathing System."

WRITER'S CRAMP.

GENERAL REMARKS ON CARRYING OUT THE EXERCISES

It is of the greatest importance that all the following movements of body and limb should, at the same time, be deep-breathing exercises, or in other words, the air should pass with a steady flow to or from the lungs in full, regular respirations. One must not hold the breath for one moment, and the next, snap after air with short asthmatic gasps. Even the smallest pause after inhalation is to be carefully avoided. When the body comes into a strained position, where further inhalation is difficult, one should immediately begin to exhale, even if the "turning point" of the movement has not quite been reached. (This applies particularly to Exercises Nos. 3, 7 and 11.)

The majority of the exercises have slow movements, and these should follow the rhythm of breathing which is most natural to the pupil when he strives to breathe with full respirations. Therefore, it is immaterial whether each respiration, or each complete movement, is counted when repeating the exercises the full number of times required. The remainder of the exercises (Nos. 2, 5, 9 and the Rubbing Exercises Nos. 16, 17 and 18) have quick movements, and here the principle is, that the pupil ultimately performs as many movements as possible to *each full respiration*. It is then easiest to count the respirations.

A complete exhalation should take a little longer time than the inhalation ; therefore, when doing slow exercises, that movement which is performed during exhalation, and which is of the same " length " as the one done during inhalation, should be performed a bit slower (this applies to Nos. 1, 6, 8 and the medium degrees of Nos. 4 and 7). In some of the other " slow " exercises the exhalation is allowed a little more movement than the inhalation (in No. 3, in advanced degrees of Nos. 4 and 7, and in many of the rubbing exercises). In the " quick " exercises, more movements are easily performed during exhalation, and one can also as a rule move the body faster during this part of the respiration ; whereas during inhalation the fast body-movements are somewhat impeded by the expanded ribs.

As a result of the first few days of exercise, parts of the body may feel tender. Every athlete has experienced these muscular "next day " or " growing pains " in arms or legs, and you will probably get the same thing round the waistline, but this need not trouble you as it will wear off if you continue. I have always felt great satisfaction in this stiffness myself, largely because I knew that the muscles which pained me were growing stronger. Still, anyone who finds the pain too severe, can rest for a day or two, or rub himself with embrocation, or some sort of liniment.

Some people might perhaps think that several of the exercises (*i.e.*, Nos. 3, 4, 5 and 7) would be more effective if performed with dumb-bells, but this is so far from being the case that I even warn against the use of them. Dumb-bells will greatly increase the common tendency to put strain in a wrong place : namely, in the muscles of the hands and arms instead of in the trunk muscles. There would also be the temptation to use the weights for pulling or swinging the body up or round, thereby making the exercise easier and of less value. I can assure you that even the strongest athlete or weight-lifter will find he gets quite sufficient vigorous exercise by performing the hardest degrees of "My System" without dumb-bells, if done correctly. Many who have tried to follow my pace in doing the exercises, soon got out of breath and none of them were able to move the trunk as quickly and powerfully as myself. There are still some people who always speak about "My System " as "light exercises," and this is true, as far as the first and easiest degrees go—which can be performed without risk or over-exertion by tiny children, delicate women and octogenarians ; but the strongest degrees are anything but "light," and will develop mighty muscles round the waistline in a short time, and by pressing very hard in the rubbing exercises, the muscles of the arms, round the shoulders and upon the breast will become highly developed.

A PROGRAMME FOR THE FIRST SIX WEEKS

All beginners, strong boys and sturdy men included, should try the easier degrees to commence with, because at first the attention should be directed chiefly to correct breathing. During very difficult movements the pupil will not easily learn the habit of breathing fully, steadily, and regularly. It should then be a rule not to attempt a strong degree, unless the previous one has been mastered and seems easy, when performed quite correctly. To do an advanced degree slovenly or wrongly does not give as great benefit to health or development as the correct carrying out of a milder degree. The best and safest way of beginning self-instruction for those in ordinary health is to follow this programme. The numbers in brackets are not the real numbers or names of the exercises, but only signify the best order of learning them, taking the easiest first.)

First Week

Study and practise :
(1) The preliminary movement " A " of Exercise No. 11 (Backward and Forward Bending of Trunk, standing).
 The special Deep-Breathing which follows each exercise.
(2) The first degree of Exercise No. 5 (Quick Arm-Circling, sitting).
(3) The first degree " A " of Exercise No. 4 (Trunk-Twisting, sitting).
(4) The preliminary movement of Exercise No. 15 (Alternate raising of Knees, with pressure, alternatively sitting).
(5) The first degree " B " of Exercise No. 4 (Sideways Trunk-Bending, sitting).
(6) The first degree of Exercise No. 8 (Body Lowering with Arm-Bending, standing).

Second Week

Add the following new exercises :
(7) The preliminary movements of Exercise No. 14 (Alternate Raising of Legs in three directions, standing).
(8) The first degree of Exercise No. 3 (Trunk-Raising, on the floor, arms assisting).
(9) The preliminary movement "A" of Exercise No. 10 (Slapping the Arms across chest, alternatively sitting).
(10) The preliminary movement "B" of Exercise No. 10 (Squatting down, feet apart and flat upon floor).
(11) The first degree of Exercise No. 6 (Single Leg-Circling, lying on the back).

53

Third Week

First degrees are, of course, omitted when second degrees are performed.
Make the following alterations:
Instead of (3), perform the second degree "B" of Exercise No. 4 (Sideways Trunk-Bending, with arm over head, standing).
Instead of (2), perform the second degree of Exercise No. 5 (Quick Arm-Circling, standing).
Add the following new exercises:
(12) The first degree of Exercise No. 7 (Trunk-Twisting with "Forward"-Leaning, sitting).
(13) The first degree of Exercise No. 2 (Quick Leg-Swinging, standing, with support).
(14) The preliminary movement of Exercise No. 13 (Trunk-Twisting sitting or standing).
(15) The preliminary movement of Exercise No. 16 (Sideways Flinging of Trunk, standing).
(16) The preliminary movement of Exercise No. 17 (Quick Trunk-Twisting with head stationary, sitting).

Fourth Week

Make the following alterations:
Instead of (3), perform the second degree "A" of Exercise No. 4 (Trunk-Twisting, with arms outstretched, standing).
Instead of (6), perform the second degree of Exercise No. 8 (Body-Lowering resting on palms and knees).
Add the following new exercises:
(17) The first degree of Exercise No. 1 (Trunk-Circling, through four points, standing).
(18) The preliminary movement of Exercise No. 12 (Sideways Trunk Bending, with alternate half Knee-Bending).
(19) The preliminary movement of Exercise No. 18 (Backward and Forward Flinging of Trunk, standing).
(20) The preliminary movement ' B ' of Exercise No. 11 (Abdominal movements, standing).

Fifth Week

Make the following alterations:
Instead of (8), perform the second degree of Exercise No. 3 (Trunk-Raising on floor or chair, hands on hips).
Instead of (11), perform the second degree of Exercise No. 6 (Lifting of stretched legs together, lying).
Instead of (12), perform the second degree of Exercise No. 7 (Trunk-Twisting with "Forward"-Leaning, arms kept outstretched, standing).
Preliminary movements are, of course, dropped when the real Rubbing Exercises are performed.
Therefore:
Combine (1) and (20) with the rubbing of Exercise No. 11 (Lengthways on front, lower back, and legs).
Combine (14) with the simplest rubbing of Exercise No. 13 (Slowly up and down the sides).

Combine (7) with the rubbing of Exercise No. 14 (Flanks and all sides of
alternately lifted legs).

Instead of (4), perform the simplest rubbing of Exercise No. 15 (Upwards
on alternately forward raised, bent legs).

Instead of (15), perform Exercise No. 16 with rubbing (Lengthways on
flanks, hips and outer side of thighs).

*These Rubbing Exercises to be studied and practised at first in some
light clothing.*

Add the following new exercise:

21) Separate neck- and foot-rubbings of Exercise No. 9. Perform first
the rubbings with the feet, then those with the hands.

Sixth Week

*Hereafter the Exercises should be performed in their right numerical
order.*

Try the following alterations:

Instead of (17), perform the second degree of Exercise No. 1 (Trunk
Circling, hands " neck rest ").

Instead of (13), perform the second degree of Exercise No. 2 (Quick Leg-
Swinging, without support).

Instead of (8), perform the third degree of Exercise No. 3 (Trunk-Raising
on floor or chair, hands " neck-rest ").

Instead of (3) and (5), perform the third degree of Exercise No. 4 (Trunk-
Twisting and Sideways Bending).

Instead of (2), perform the third degree of Exercise No. 5 (Quick Arm-
Circling with long lunge).

Instead of (11), perform the third degree of Exercise No. 6 (Circling of
both legs simultaneously, lying).

Instead of (12), perform the third degree of Exercise No. 7 (Trunk-
Twisting in the positions of leaning over alternate hips).

Instead of (6), perform the third degree of Exercise No. 8 (Body-
Lowering, resting on palms and toes).

Combine the neck- and foot-rubbings of Exercise No. 9 (21).

Instead of the slapping (9), perform the rubbing of Exercise No. 10
(arms, shoulders, and round armpits); but keep up the
Squatting (10) as a special exercise until it can be combined
with the rubbing.

Combine (18) with the simplest rubbing of Exercise No. 12 (up the thighs
and hips alternately, and across abdomen).

Combine (16) with the rubbing of Exercise No. 17 (across breast, slowly
at first).

Combine (19) with the rubbing of Exercise No. 18 (up abdomen, down
the loins).

If not too cold, the rubbings learned in the foregoing week are now
performed stripped, and after another week of practice, *all* the Rubbing
Exercises are performed without any clothing.

It depends, of course, entirely on the ability and strength of the
student when the still stronger degrees of the first eight exercises and
the more elaborate additions to several of the rubbing exercises can be
mastered.

Very weak or elderly persons should spread this programme over
twelve weeks or more, and should in many cases never advance to the
most difficult or strenuous forms of the exercises.

THE BEST HOURS FOR DOING THE EXERCISES

and their proper sequence when learnt

There are two or three times of day which are suitable for perform-ing these exercises ; namely, when the clothes are being changed for any reason. (1) In the morning (before breakfast) ; (2) when home from business (before dinner or supper) ; and (3) when going to bed.

The normal way is to do the first eight exercises (do not take breakfast or a cup of tea in bed !) in your pyjamas or a jersey (if you want to reduce fat, or if you feel the cold very much, wear a sweater) ; then take the bath and rough towelling, finishing up with the ten rubbing exercises. If preferred, the bath can be taken first, then the rubbing exercises, and when partly dressed the " first eight " exercises. This plan may be a good one if you are accustomed to jump straight into your bath from the bed ; but it is not so good if the eight exercises make you perspire, in your clothes. In that case it is better to do all the exercises stripped, performing alternately a rubbing and an ordinary exercise in the following order : The bath, Exercises Nos. 11, 10, 1, 12, 2, 13, 3, 14, 4, 15, 5, 16, 6, 17, 7, 18, 8 and 9. This alternate sequence is also the most comfortable in very warm weather ; but then you should naturally take the bath at the very end of the procedure, owing to your probably heavy perspiration.

The whole " System " performed in the morning will give the average healthy individual a feeling of physical buoyancy and good conscience for the day, but for rather weak or very busy people it is better to divide the " System " into two, or even three parts, to be performed at the above-mentioned practical hours, for five to ten minutes each time. When dividing up into parts you may follow your own course, or the first eight exercises can, for instance, be performed in the morning, with bath before or after, and then the rubbing exercises in the evening before going to bed.

Should it be found that this causes disturbed slumber, a different time should be chosen first of all, but later on, when the nerves have grown steadier and stronger, you will sleep the better for your evening exercise, supposing you do not take a late supper. It should be remem-bered, when the rubbing exercises are taken by themselves, always to begin with No. 11 and finish with No. 9. These ten rubbing exercises with deep breathing during and in between them, take but a bare seven minutes to go through, yet the result is that you lie down in bed with a delightful feeling all over the skin, and fairly certain of a good night's rest. No one ought to deny himself these seven minutes, especially during cold weather.

Exercise should not be indulged in too soon after a meal. A child may do it without harm, but a grown-up should let at least one-and-a-half hours elapsed after the last meal, and if there is a tendency to indigestion, two full hours.

Some people take two baths daily, viz., a cold douche in the morning and a warm or hot bath when coming home from business. This is a splendid plan, and they might arrange to do some of the exercises with each bath.

I think the reader will understand that it is not necessary for a water bath to immediately precede the rubbing exercises, as, when stripped, these exercises form in themselves an air bath.

While learning, the time used in doing all the eighteen exercises will be about twenty-five to thirty minutes, on account of the necessary reference to the text or illustrations. If more time is spent, then the pauses of "thinking" are really too long. When the pupil is thoroughly conversant with the "System," however, the whole series can be easily performed in twenty minutes, with bath included. And extraordinarily strong and practised individuals can do it in exactly fifteen minutes, as I personally have proved more than 1,400 times at public demonstrations (400 times in Great Britain).

The "slow" exercises must never be hurried, but the "quick" ones must, of course, be done very quickly in order to make this fifteen minutes' performance possible.

The whole "System" being known by heart, unnecessary pauses are never made. Each exercise ends by an exhalation, during the last part of which one takes up the position of the next exercise—or of the special deep-breathings when such are wanted—so that the following inhalation naturally forms part of the next exercise. Thus the whole series "flows" steadily and uninterruptedly, disturbed neither by fussiness nor hesitation.

The rubbing exercises, Nos. 9 to 18, form a small "System" in themselves; but it is wrong to confine oneself to the Exercises Nos. 1 to 8, which I know some people do. They will surely miss some quick trunk movements, and a deep knee-bending as well, and some knee-bendings (see page 60 of the volume in hand).

DESCRIPTION OF THE EXERCISES

Deep-Breathing Exercises

To stand up and without any physical exertion take long breaths—as is often recommended, especially in German books—is unnatural and absurd, in fact may positively cause derangement in the relative pressure of the vessels of the body, and produce giddiness. When you intend to breathe deeply, a need for more air should be felt, for which reason these same exercises are suitable only during or after a corresponding exertion of the body, while they, at the same time, have the important task of re-establishing the regular beating of the heart.

In the former editions of " My System," a particular " Respiratory pause " was described, to be strictly observed after every exercise. But now that all exercises are at the same time breathing exercises, it is no longer so necessary always to observe such regular pauses.

Only beginners and weak persons, for whom even the easiest degrees can be difficult, need make regular use of the respiratory pause. Whereas, advanced persons will often feel no need for it after the "slow" exercises. More deep-breathings may then be taken after the "quick" exercises (Nos. 2, 5, 16, 17 and 18), and after the somewhat hard No. 8, immediately preceding the bath.

During the respiratory pauses the performer should stand quite still in a comfortable position with hands on hips, and endeavour to inspire and expire the largest possible quantity of air.

I do not, therefore, now recommend carrying out of " accompanying" movements such as arm-raising, heels-raising and knee-bendings, because it is my experience that such movements are apt to distract the attention from the main object, namely, the movements of the chest itself.

In the Swedish Drill, it is true, the only " breathing exercise " s composed of just raising the arms for inhaling and lowering them for exhaling, and no instructions at all are given as to how the air is to come in and out of the lungs. But that it is a sad delusion to believe, that we expire the air simply by lowering the arms, anyone can convince himself by the following experiment : Stand with arms hanging loosely by the sides, and take a full breath ; then lift the arms slowly sideways, at the same time performing deep exhalation. If the person exercising has even a little bit of control over the breathing muscles, he will find that the exhalation can be equally thorough, whether the arms move up or down or hang relaxed by the sides.

As I have written a complete book on how one should breathe under all conditions (" My Breathing System "),* it is hardly necessary to give long explanations here. I will, therefore, confine myself to giving a few practical hints.

* Published by Athletic Publications, Ltd. 3s. 6d. net.

The ideal thing is to get as much air as possible in and out, with the least muscular effort, and, if it is a matter of strenuous or quick exercises, then in addition, in the shortest possible time. But even if the respirations in the latter case are fairly quick ones, they should always be quite full, never shallow. Learn to move the lower ribs sideways, and also to "lengthen" the chest straight upwards like a concertina which is pulled out, by one handle being held up, the other down. The arms should help in this movement, the hands pressing upon the hip bones in a downward direction. A vacuum will thus be created, into which the air will rush of its own accord. The air then should not be drawn in by using the nose as a suction pump. The nose should only be a *passive* passage and that both for the inhaled and exhaled air.

The nostrils must, of course, be kept wide open, but if there is only a narrow passage for the air at the root of the nose or roof of the mouth, one should get a surgeon to remove the obstructions.

The old-fashioned Swedish "Deep Breathing" method with arching of the chest, pressing back of elbows and shoulders, and drawing in of the abdomen, must be quite condemned. It is a frightful strain of the muscles which does not give much air to the lungs. There is really a hollow created between the shoulder-blades, so that the air-space in the lungs does not increase, but is only shifted.

Expiration simply takes place by relaxing the inspiratory muscles, so that the chest falls together by its own weight and drives the air out through the nose. If there is time to do so, exhalation can be made deeper still by the contraction of the lower ribs, performed by the small muscles placed between and under those ribs ; or quite mechanically by pressing the ribs together with the palms of the hands. But do not on any account draw the abdomen in, as the ribs then cannot properly contract, and even if the diaphragm, in that case, presses some air out of the lower lobes of the lungs, their greater portion will not be emptied of air. The abdominal muscles should in other words be left relaxed both during inhalation and exhalation, so as not to hinder the full but easy respiration. That frightful habit, characteristic of so many military men, and so-called "Gymnasts," continually to draw the abdomen in, rigid and contracted (" muscle-bound "), is to blame for many digestive troubles in that all internal movements and "massage" are strangled. Yes ! there is absolutely not enough room left for the organs to function properly. These people use the abdominal muscles to support the skeleton and balance the body, instead of using the muscles of the flanks and back. It is wrong to have a weak, distended abdominal wall, which is incapable of withstanding the pressure from the heavy internal organs. It is equally wrong to be " hollow " in this part of the anatomy. For the common superstition that such " hollow-ness " is beautiful and healthy, the " smart " reproductions as per example in our authorised Drill Manuals, are largely to blame. By visiting a museum and studying an antique statue of an athlete in profile, one will at once realise that the ideal of beauty and a natural carriage of the body demands that the abdomen shall at least protrude as much as the chest. It is quite possible to have a straight back without looking like a pouter-pigeon.

Correct breathing is almost noiseless. Should one therefore hear oneself snuffing or blowing, one knows that there is something wrong. If one is deaf, one must let oneself be controlled by a friend. If the respiration be noisy, it is a proof that the air passage is narrowed, as per example : the wind blowing through an open door is hardly heard ; on the other hand, when the door is shut, it whistles and howls through the creaks and keyhole.

There is nothing artificial about the breathing method which I recommend here. It is the only natural and right one, which should be employed, not only during my exercises, but also during daily life, immediately on undertaking any body-movement. For example, during walking and cycling, one can take three or four paces or treads during inhalation, and five or six during exhalation. It will only be necessary to count for a week or two, as it will soon become an unconscious habit, so that the chest will hereafter work in this complete way, without wasting any thought on the matter.

Synopsis :
Each of the deep respirations consists of a very full inhalation through the nose, and a deep, steady exhalation also through the nose. Place the hands on the hips, the elbows well out, not forced backwards. The rules for inhalation are (see Fig. 1) :

    1. Distend the nostrils and move the lower ribs as far as possible outwards.
    2. Stretch the whole upper part of the trunk.
    3. Do not arch the upper chest into a cramped position.
    4. Keep the abdomen naturally relaxed.

And the rules for exhalation (see Fig. 2) :

    1. Let the ribs and the whole upper part of the trunk sink down.
    2. Draw the lower ribs inwards, and together as much as possible.
    3. Keep the abdomen naturally relaxed.

Common faults in this deep breathing are : during *inhalation*—drawing the abdomen inwards, bending the head too far backwards, forcing the shoulders back instead of lifting them, sucking the air into the nose with a loud noise so that the nostrils are partly closed ; during *exhalation*—bending the body too much forwards instead of contracting the chest, keeping the abdomen fixed or drawn inwards, breathing the air out forcibly through the mouth. In " My Breathing System " I have scientifically proved that exhalation through the mouth after nasal inhalation—which unfortunately is still often taught—is absolutely wrong.

Knee-Bending Exercises

Whereas it is not advisable to perform heel-raising and full knee-bending during the respiratory pauses, even for the strongest individuals, it is in many instances an excellent plan to carry out these powerful leg movements—as a special exercise that can easily be performed just before or after Ex. No. 8. It is particularly recommended to motorists and others, who are too lazy, or who don't take time to walk. I will here describe a slow and a quick exercise, both only for advanced performers.

    1.—Raise yourself slowly up on the toes, with heels together, at the same time lifting the arms sideways and pressing the hands backwards at the wrists, with fingers well stretched, all the while inhaling (see Fig. 3). Lower the body slowly while bending the legs, knees well out-

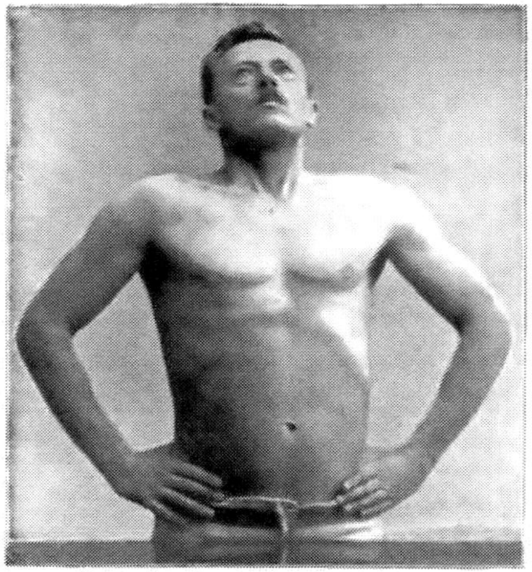

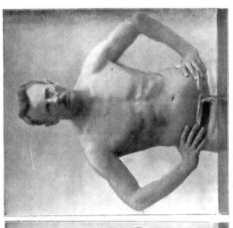

FIG. 1.—THE CORRECT POSE FOR INHALATION, FRONT VIEW

FIG. 2.—THE CORRECT POSE FOR INHALATION, FRONT VIEW

Note the difference in the triangles formed by the nipples and navel

wards, until the seat touches the heels. The arms should simultaneously be lowered to the inside of the knees, with fingers clenched and fists turned inwards from the wrist, during expiration (see Fig. 4). Then the legs and fingers are once more straightened while the arms are lifted and you must take up the previously described "stretched" position, and again bend the knees as before ; repeat this ten times up and ten times down during ten full respirations ; breathing in always during the upward movement, and out during the downward movement. During the last expiration, just lower the heels and arms very slowly.

2.—You should perform similar full knee-bendings, but now as quickly as possible; after, practise two bendings and stretchings during inhalation, and three double movements during exhalation. The heels remain raised and well pressed together all through, as in the first exercise. There are no finger and wrist movements, nor arm raising and lowering. The arms are held out obliquely in front or inclined to sides to balance the body. Perform up to twenty knee-bendings during four full respirations, but don't forget to stretch the legs completely in each upward movement

Relaxation Exercises

Muscles increase in strength, quickness and endurance by quick changes between work and rest. One should therefore be capable of completely relaxing or slackening the muscles, either *all* at once, when the body rests, or during a particular movement; slacken all those that are not in use while the movement is in progress. The faulty principles in School, Army and many Home Systems of physical culture, have caused the majority of people to be more or less stiff in the muscles, or "muscle-bound." One ought then to give oneself a course in muscle-relaxation.

Sit on a chair, letting the left arm hang quite limp by the side. Then feel its muscles with the fingers of the right hand, and convince yourself that they are quite soft. Now take hold of the left wrist and lift the left arm up to shoulder height. Be careful, that you really lift the whole weight of the left arm with the right, as the left arm must not help itself to be raised, and must of course not resist. Suddenly release your grip, and let the arm fall. It should then dangle to and fro before coming to rest in a vertical position. Repeat same exercise with relaxed right arm. In a like manner then lift a leg with both hands and let it drop ; or lie down on the floor and ask a friend to lift and release the legs, one after the other. The neck can be exercised in the same manner, although it is harder to relax, but be careful that the head drops on to a soft cushion. The abdominal muscles are best relaxed in a sitting position, leaning well back, or when lying in bed. The best time for carrying out these exercises is, then, just before going to sleep.

Convince yourself that the whole body and every limb rests on its particular part of the bed with the whole of its weight ; in other words, try to make yourself as heavy as you can. Then you will be more sure to get healthy and refreshing sleep.

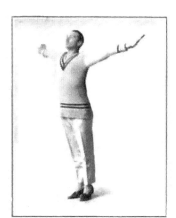

Fig. 3.

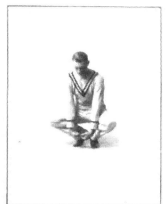

Fig. 4.

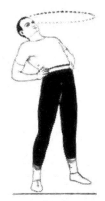

Fig. 5.

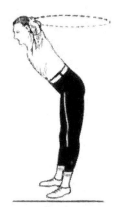

Fig. 6.

64

EXERCISE No. 1

Slow Trunk-Circling

This exercise is put first in the " System," because, when carried out in its original form (third degree, see Figs. 7-10), it is excellent for thoroughly stretching the whole body when one has jumped out of bed in the morning. As it is, however, somewhat difficult to perform correctly by beginners, these should not immediately tackle it, but ought, during the first weeks, to follow the programme set out on page 52.

First Degree

Stand with feet astride, hands on hips (" hips firm "), with thumbs to the rear. Bend the upper part of the body to the left, from the hips, then backwards (see Fig. 5), next to the right, then to the front, while the seat is pushed out backwards, and finally to the left again. Here one has the four points which the trunk should pass when one begins to circle it round. As will be seen, the exercise is a combination of sideways bending and forward-backward leaning ; whereas turning or twisting of the body must not take place here. The body should therefore continually face the same front, that is forward, during the whole exercise. All movement should take place in the waist, while the head is held steadily in a natural position. It is recommended to let the eyes rest on a point straight to the front and slightly raised. To let them roll round from floor to ceiling and walls makes the correct carrying out of the exercise impossible and brings forth dizziness. Be careful not to bend the back during the forward leaning; it should be quite straight with the abdomen distended. As soon as the four positions have been mastered, especially the rather difficult forward leaning, begin to "round off " these " corners," in that the body swings round steadily in circles, first five times one way, and then five the other. The movement must be suited to the full respiration; inspiration during the back half of each " circle " and expiration during the forward half.

Second Degree

Hands at " neck rest," elbows well back, which is difficult during the forward half of the circle. Body movements and breathing same as First Degree. Don't drop the head and elbows or curve the back when leaning forward ! (Fig. 6.)

Third Degree

The arms are held well stretched upwards, touching the ears, the hands folded and wrists bent at right angles to the forearm (Figs. 7-10). The arms are still held tight to the head during forward leaning ; it is a

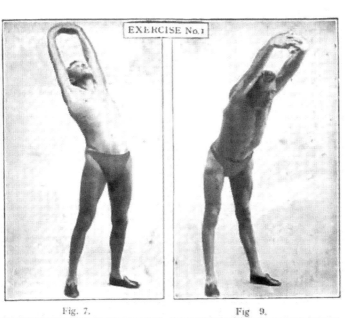

EXERCISE No. 1

Fig. 7.

Fig. 9.

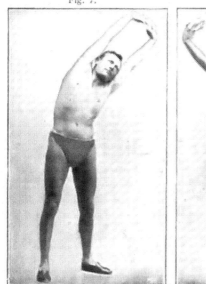

Fig. 8.

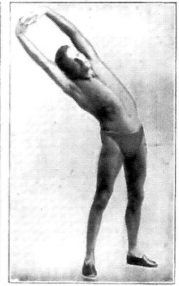

Fig. 10.

common mistake to swing them round in the shoulder joints. Remember it is the muscles round the waist that should move the trunk, with head, arms and hands as dead weight

FOURTH DEGREE

Same movements as in preceding degree, but as one's breathing is now deeper, one may inhale during one complete circle and exhale during the next. Either let the inhalation circle go a little faster, or let the inhalation take three-fourths of a circle and the exhalation one-fourth.

EXERCISE No. 2

Quick Leg-Swinging

FIRST DEGREE

Support yourself with one hand on a fixed piece of furniture or a door-handle and put the other on the hip. (Should you be suffering from weakness of the legs, then you can also support yourself with this hand, say, on the back of a chair.)

Swing the one leg like a pendulum, forward and backward from the hip-joint. It must be held as straight as a cork leg in the knee-joint. This is easiest to perform if the toes are pointed upwards. If you stand sideways on to a looking-glass, it will be noticed that the leg which you thought was straight will often give way considerably in the knee. Even if to begin with, you do not swing the leg very fast you should still see that there is not the least pause in the movements. These swings with straight leg are quite short (30 to 40 degrees), but are finished with some very long swings when the foot is kicked high up fore and aft, in order to loosen the joints. During these finishing-swings the leg must be limp with all muscles relaxed, and the knee may be bent. When the hip-joint is made more flexible, the foot can reach higher up than the head (see Fig. 11).

The exercise should stretch itself over four full respirations, the long swings being performed during the last one. Thereafter repeat exercise with other leg. Beginners often have difficulty with breathing steadily, i.e., independently of the quick movements. They are inclined either to breathe short, in time with the swings, or to hold the breath. To get hold of the right method, you can for example stand still, while filling the lungs completely, and then when commencing to exhale slowly, swing the leg quickly and count the number of swings you can perform before all air is out of the lungs.

SECOND DEGREE

Both hands " hips firm," or arms hanging loosely by the sides. This makes it additionally a balancing exercise. As you grow stronger and more practised, the movement is performed much faster, so that a great number of swings to each respiration will be possible, as you also learn to breathe deeper. You can then diminish the number of respira-

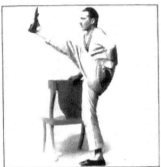

Fig. 11.

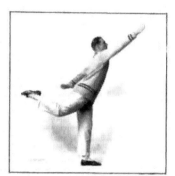

Fig. 12.

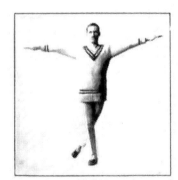

Fig. 13.

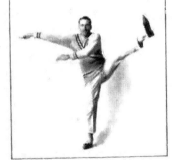

Fig. 14.

These photos and several of the others are of the Author's
eldest son, Ib, at the age of 22, 34 and 37 years

tions until at last two will suffice for a score of short swings and two long ones with each leg. During the latter, the arms should be swung loosely in time with the leg. When the leg goes forward and up, the corresponding arm is swung as far as possible backward, the other arm simultaneously forward, and vice versa (Fig. 12). It is particularly the muscles of the hips, flanks and lower back that are strengthened by correct carrying out of this exercise.

THIRD DEGREE

This is a more difficult balancing exercise. The arms are held outstretched to the sides, with fingers straight and palms down. While breathing in and out once, the leg is swung sideways (alternately to right and left) *behind* the other, in short swings (Fig. 13). During the next respiration it is swung sideways in front of the other leg, in short swings, during inhalation, and in long, " loose " ones during exhalation In conjunction with the latter long swings, both arms are thrust to the same side, always opposite to the leg (Fig. 14). These arm-swings then resemble those in use during a spurt on speed skates. Hereafter repeat with other leg.

FOURTH DEGREE

A combination of the two preceding. During first inhalation : short forward-backward swings with left leg. During first exhalation : long forward-backward swings with left leg and both arms. Second respiration : the same is repeated with right leg. Third inhalation : short side-swings with left leg behind right, arms outstretched sideways. Third exhalation : long side-swings with left leg in front of right, arms swung as described in third degree. Fourth respiration : similar swings with right leg.

EXERCISE No. 3

Slow Trunk-Raising and Lowering

FIRST DEGREE

Lay yourself on your back in front of a heavy piece of furniture and put the front third of your feet underneath (a little more than the toes). Should there be no room here, then pull half out the bottom drawer and put the feet under ; or remove it altogether and put your feet in the opening. The knees are bent the more, the lower the space is for the feet, as the ankle might otherwise be overstrained. If no suitable furniture be available, you can fasten a pair of straps to the floor or wall, as the feet *must* have support, otherwise the exercise is valueless. In this position, flat on the back, all muscles of the neck, shoulders and back should be relaxed, so as to really rest in comfort. Thereupon fill the lungs completely, and just after commencing the exhalation, raise the body to the forward-leaned sitting position, by means of pulling with the feet and using the abdominal muscles. So as not to strain these in the beginning, you may help with elbows and hands, which are pressed against the floor, and carried backward as the body rises. It is a bad mistake to raise oneself with a jerk, or push, with head and

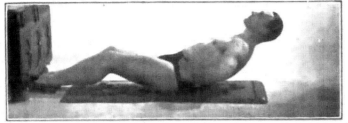

Fig. 15

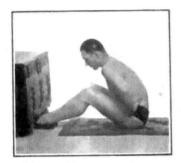

Fig. 16.

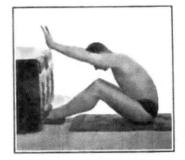

Fig. 17.

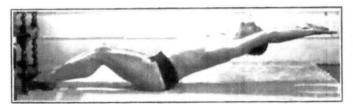

Fig. 18.

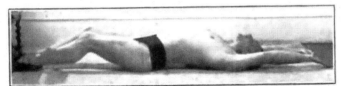

Fig. 19.

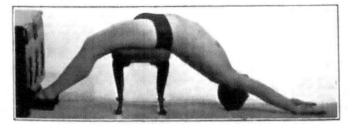

Fig. 20.

shoulders, or to roll the body up. The head's natural position is maintained while the whole upper body is moved in one piece with the hipjoint as axis of rotation. Don't stick the chin out, duck the head or draw in the abdomen, when the body is leant forward. Rather seek to distend the stomach between the knees. The exhalation is performed during this body-lifting and without any pause you immediately commence to lower the body backwards and to inhale. As the body nears the floor and the abdominal muscles gradually contract, you will hardly be able to get more air. Instead of committing the error of holding the breath, you should immediately commence exhalation and finish the same lying on the floor. During the body lowering you also use the hands and elbows as supports ; but refrain from throwing the head or eyes back or bend the chin on to the chest. While in the resting position fill the lungs completely once more, then raise the body the second time, but just beforehand begin to exhale. If you don't do this you will run the risk of holding your breath during the body-raising. As will be seen, there belong two complete respirations to each perfected movement, up and down. Perform six such double movements and increase these to a dozen in a few weeks.

SECOND DEGREE

" Hips firm," as shown in Figs. 15 and 16. Now there is no rest pause on the floor ; but the body is moved steadily and slowly up and down almost in beat with the natural full respiration. To avoid the least pause in the breathing one should begin the exhalation a moment before the change of direction of movement (but be careful not to shorten the movements!). So one inhales during the greater part of the body-lowering, and exhales during the latter part of it *and* during the whole of the rising. To sit on a stool, or sideways on a chair, while doing the exercise gives more movement to the waist without being harder ; it soon becomes more comfortable. On reaching right down all the trunk muscles should relax, so that the body hangs like a dead weight, with the forehead near the floor (compare Fig. 20).

THIRD DEGREE

" Neck rest." Movement and respiration as in Second Degree. When carried out on the floor, the elbows must touch same, and during the rising should maintain their " back " position. Sitting on a stool, it is also wrong to give a jerk with elbows and head in order to rise.

FOURTH DEGREE

On the floor or a chair, as shown in Figs. 17-20. The arms are held quietly stretched up beside the ears, as in a dive into water, and are so used as an extra weight for the abdominal muscles to lift, during their steady contraction. To throw the arms forward quite spoils the value of this Exercise. Even to raise them and bring them forwards sooner than the trunk is a serious mistake. They should be kept close to the ears the whole time.

EXERCISE No. 4

Slow Trunk-Twisting with Sideways-Bending

FIRST DEGREE

To be sure of a correct performance of this exercise in the beginning, it is best to do the twisting and sideways-bending separately.

A. Sit on a chair (either on the front edge of the seat, or use one without a back), and twist one or both legs round the legs of the chair whereby the lower body is made unmovable. Or you may simply sit down on the floor. With hands at " hips firm," the upper part of the body is turned slowly, but without pauses alternately, as far as possible to right and left, the head following the body movements. Inhale one way and exhale the opposite. Compare Fig. 104, illustrating a similar movement, but with head stationary.

When four and a half double movements with four and a half full respirations are completed, a pause is held in the twisted position, an exhalation being taken. Thereafter five similar double twistings are performed, but the breathing is now, of course, done the opposite way as was the case before, *i.e.*, if you inhaled to the right before, you should now exhale to this side and inhale to the left.

B. Sit on a chair, arms hanging down limp. Bend the upper part of the body slowly, but without pausing, as far as possible to right and left alternately. Try every time to reach the floor with your finger tips. You may also bend the head. Inhale one way and exhale the other. Perform nineteen movements during ten full respirations, and do not forget to change the breathing when half-way is reached, in exactly the same way as explained in "*A*." It is even more important here, so as not to develop the chest one-sidedly.

SECOND DEGREE

It is still recommended to perform the twisting and sideways bending apart.

A. Stand with the feet as much as possible apart and parallel, or still better, with the toes a trifle inwards. The arms raised sideways with fingers lightly closed, not clenched. The trunk is twisted alternately to right and left as in first degree, but now that the seat and hips no longer are held firm by sitting down, it is harder to limit the movement to the waist. One is likely to move the feet, twist round in the knees, or to only turn the head, whereby, of course, the benefit to the important organs in the abdominal cavity is *nil*. One should therefore fix the hips (keep them squarely to the front the whole time), or, still better, push forward the left hip whenever the left shoulder goes back, and control the right side of the body in the same way every time its turn comes. The head follows the body's movements. The arms must not swing the body round; they are held still, but not stiff, and are moved together with the upper part of the body and the head, as a dead weight alone by the effort of the muscles around the waist. The movement is illustrated by Figs. 22 and 23, but the feet should be much more apart. The breathing, with change half-way, and the number of

repetitions is the same as in the First Degree. But do not forget to start
the first inhalation while the arms are raised. If the position of the
arms tires you, just lower them with each exhalation.

B. Stand with heels together, and bend alternately to the sides as
in First Degree, but each time one bends to the right, the left arm, half
bent and with palm downward, is brought across the head, thereby increasing that weight which acts on the flank muscles (see Fig. 21). So
also every time one bends to the left, the right arm forms a similar arch
over the head. The breathing, with change in the middle of the exercise, and number of repetitions as in First Degree.

THIRD DEGREE

Combination of the twisting and sideways-bending. Each time the
upper part of the body has been turned round to one of those positions
described in " A " of Second Degree, for instance Fig. 22, it is slowly bent
right down sideways, so that the closed fist touches the floor between the
feet (Fig. 24), and is immediately brought back again to the upright
position (Fig. 22). It is then twisted right round to the other side
(Fig. 23), and bent fully down till the other hand touches the floor
(Fig. 25), and so on. To begin with, one can bend the knee that corresponds with the arm that is down, to make it easier, but as one becomes
more pliable above the hips, both knees remain straight. Do not turn
the head and look down—there must be no marked movement in the
neck, either in the shoulders or arms ; all movement is concentrated in
the waist-line, the muscles of which move the whole upper body steadily
and slowly, without jerks or swings. The separate movements of this
combined exercise must be clearly marked, but without pauses be performed continuously. Otherwise the regularity of the respirations will
be interfered with. One inhales coming up and going half-way round,
and exhales during remainder of turning and going down. Ten such
triple movements during ten full respirations.

After sufficient practice the feet may be placed less apart. If now
the hand cannot reach the floor unless the knee is bent, the reason is
simply that the twist has been made in the legs and not in the waist,
and the hip-bone will then hinder the sideways-bending.

FOURTH DEGREE

Here a short double sideways-bending is added. Begin for instance
with the left hand touching the floor (Fig. 25). Then raise the upper
body (Fig. 23) and twist round to the left (Fig. 22). Instead of now
going right down to the right, you should only bend half-way, as shown
in the dotted lines of Fig. 26, then quickly up again and as far as possible
over to the left (i.e., " backwards " as seen from the hips point of view,
as shown in the full lines of Fig. 26). You can naturally not go very far
this way. To end up with, you then—without any pause—perform
the whole sideways-bending to the right, until the right hand touches
the floor (Fig. 24). Thereupon a similar five-double movement the
opposite way. You should now inhale while coming up and twisting
right round, and exhale during the two short and the long " sideways "
bendings. Ten five-double movements during ten full respirations.

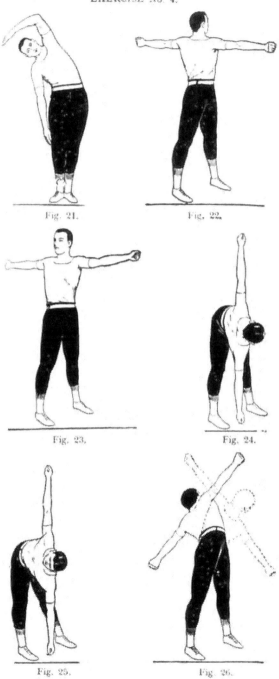

Fig. 21.

Fig. 22.

Fig. 23.

Fig. 24.

Fig. 25.

Fig. 26.

EXERCISE No. 5

Quick Arm-Circling

FIRST DEGREE

Sit on the chair (preferably a stool), and raise the arms sideways with fingers together and stretched straight, palms upward. Then swing both arms fairly fast round in small circles (of 12 inches in diameter); upward in the front half and downward in the back half (compare Fig. 27). Thereupon each arm is swung separately, loosely and in as large circles as possible. Be careful to get the arm well back and near to the ear. As many small circles as possible are performed during three full respirations; while during a fourth respiration, the one arm be swung in large circles, and during the fifth the other arm. The exercise is thereafter repeated with small and large circles in opposite directions, likewise during five full respirations. The palms are now turned down, and the arms are moved downwards in the front half of the circle, and upwards in rear half (compare Fig. 29). If you find it difficult to breathe naturally and deeply during these fast arm-movements, you may try this way. Fill the lungs completely and then see how many times you can swing the arms while you are letting the air slowly out through the nose.

SECOND DEGREE

This is carried out standing, with one foot slightly in front of the other (see Fig. 27). Arm-circling and breathing as in First Degree in addition to which one now circles both arms together during the large swings (Fig. 28). Put the other foot in front when the arms are swung in opposite direction. Be careful to force the arms well back while describing the circles. A common fault in the small circles is to move the hands up and down only, instead of in real circles. Do not forget to keep the arms absolutely limp during the large circles.

THIRD DEGREE

With a long forward lunge, bending front knee, straight line from head to rear foot (Figs. 29 and 30), arm circling and breathing as before, but the small circles are now done very quickly, so that a greater number is performed, especially during the expirations; you may then gradually limit the exercise to six full respirations in all. Change feet when half way in the exercise.

FOURTH DEGREE

Lunge and arm circling as in preceding degree. The body is now twisted slowly round from the waist (with arms still circling rapidly) alternately to right and left, and in beat with the full, steady respiration. Inhalation takes place every time the chest is turned towards the side of the straight and rear leg (Fig. 31), exhalation when it is turned towards the side of the bent leg (Fig. 32). In other words, one breathes in the one way and out the other. The large loose swings are only performed during the last exhalation of each series (not during the whole third respiration): the twisting ceases and the large swings are done while facing to the front.

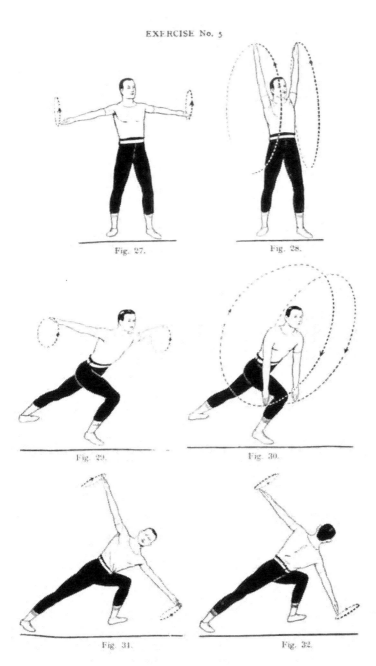

Fig. 27.

Fig. 28.

Fig. 29.

Fig. 30.

Fig. 31.

Fig. 32.

EXERCISE No. 6

Slow Leg-Circling

FIRST DEGREE

Lie flat on your back with hands at "neck-rest," and move the straight left leg slowly round in circles of about 30 ins. diameter (see Fig. 33). The leg should not be lifted much more than 45° from the floor. Inhale every time the leg is raised, exhale during the downward movement. When six such circles have been completed, two circles as large as possible should be performed (Fig. 34). As the foot (with toes pointed) is carried sideways, the elbows should steady the body by pressing against the floor, so preventing it from rolling over. Thereafter eight corresponding circles with the right leg during eight full respirations. Then the left leg is again moved round slowly but in the opposite direction to which it was first moved. To finish with, the right leg is circled similarly.

SECOND DEGREE

Take a deep inhalation while resting on the floor. During the following exhalation, lift both stretched legs to a height of 45° from the floor, and lower at once (Fig. 37). This movement is repeated eight times during eight full respirations in that one lies with the majority of one's muscles relaxed every time one inhales.

THIRD DEGREE

The legs, perfectly straight and with pointed toes, are circled slowly the same as in First Degree, only both simultaneously (Fig. 38). In the small circles the legs and feet are pressed hard together each time they meet (Fig. 35), each leg thus describing the letter "D," or its reflection. In the large circles the one leg must of course give way to the other, like the blades of a pair of scissors, so that both on crossing one another can move right round without interruption (Fig. 36). The head may be lifted a little so that one can see whether it is done correctly. As before, eight circles in each direction, but the whole exercise now only lasts the time of 16 respirations, therefore, only half the time of the First Degree. The feet may in the beginning rest for a moment upon the floor after each circuit. The legs and insteps should be kept straight also in the large circles.

FOURTH DEGREE

Ten small and two large circles in each direction. The heels should just touch the floor after each completed circle, but not rest upon it. The movement is now done very slowly with the breathing equally deep. The task for the abdominal muscles is also increased by wearing heavy boots. The head rests on the floor and the hands are put flat under the hollow of the back, or in the position of "hips firm," or they may be stretched up past the ears and touch the ground beyond the head. Another way of doing the fourth degree is to keep the stretched legs pressed together continuously while swinging them slowly round in as wide circles as possible, six times in each direction. To prevent the body from rolling over, the arms are kept sideways with palms pressing against the floor.

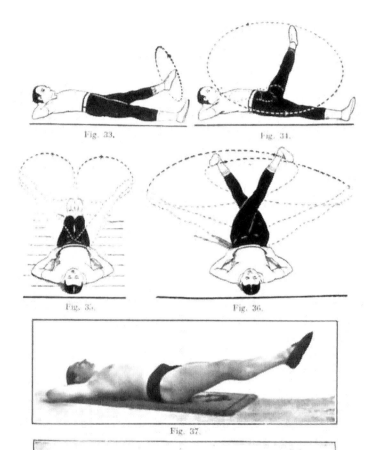

Fig. 33.

Fig. 34.

Fig. 35.

Fig. 36.

Fig. 37.

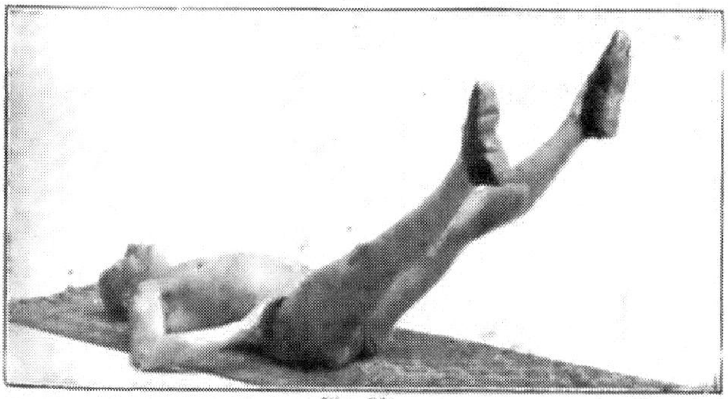

Fig. 38.

EXERCISE No. 7

Slow Trunk-Twisting with " Forward "-Leaning

FIRST DEGREE

Sit on a chair or stool, with legs gripping those of the chair, as in First Degree, A, of Exercise No. 4. While inhaling, raise the arms slowly sideways to shoulder height with fists closed lightly and the arm muscles relaxed. Only the shoulders' effort should lift the arms. During exhalation, and while lowering the arms, twist the upper body round to the left (in the waist line, keeping hips and seat fixed), and then lean it slowly " forward," that is over the left hip (see Fig. 39). This must be done without lowering the chin or rounding the back. When all the air is exhaled, another inhalation takes place during which the following movements will be performed : The upper part of the body is raised, with simultaneous arm-lifting, and then twisted back again to the front. During the immediately following deep exhalation the movements that were carried out to the left are now done in exactly the same manner to the right, and so on continuously, always with inhalation while rising and turning to the front, and exhalation while turning to either right or left side and leaning. 10 complete movements during 10 respirations.

When after some practice one is able to twist the body in the waist and not in the knees, the movements are carried out standing, with legs wide apart, as in Exercise No. 4, Second Degree, A. As the upper body is leant over the hip the back should be slightly hollowed and the eyes looking somewhat upwards (Fig. 40).

SECOND DEGREE

This is always performed standing. Breathing and body movements as in First Degree, whereas the arms are now continually held sideways in shoulder height and the feet less apart. The movements are steady and continuous, in that you (with the exception of the preliminary inhalation with arms lifting) inhale every time the trunk is raised and during first half of the twisting ; and exhale during the latter's second half and during the leaning over the hip. Only if you have neither got the lungs completely filled nor emptied, should small pauses be held, in the front-facing position or leaning to the side. The succession of the positions of this exercise is as follows : Figs. 22 (see Exercise No. 4), 41, 22, 23, 43, 23, 22, 41 and so on.

THIRD DEGREE

The preliminary movement is the same as in the Second Degree ; during the first inhalation raise the arms slowly, then while exhaling twist the body round to the left (Fig. 22), and lean it over the left hip (Fig. 41). Then instead of returning to the vertical position before twisting to the right, you should now twist completely round in the leaning position, at the same time inhaling. The upper body therefore remains in the inclined position (i.e. retains its angle), but the chest is now uppermost (Fig. 42). Following this twist, and during exhalation, the trunk is raised slowly and without pausing, leaned " forward " (that

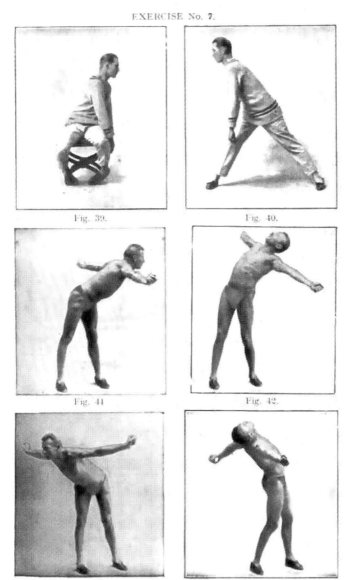

Fig. 39.

Fig. 40.

Fig. 41

Fig. 42.

Fig. 43.

Fig. 44.

is, to the original right) over the right hip (Fig. 43) ; over which a similar twist, but now to the left, takes place while inhaling (Fig. 44). This exercise thus falls into a measure of two beats only. The one is perpetually a complete turning of the trunk, and the other a raising and " forward " leaning to alternate sides. Do not bend the knees more than you can help, and the hips and legs should, as far as possible, retain their fixed front all the while. The head and arms should not be forced much backwards, although the back is continually held a little hollowed. It is the muscles of the waist that should move the upper body steadily. At every twist the arms come round passing the vertical plane, so that the one hand points to the ceiling, and its shoulder is pressed back, the other hand having pointed to the floor. A common mistake is to lean too far downwards so that the correct angle cannot be maintained during the twist that follows. It is really only when one has wrongly turned the hips away from the front that this new mistake so easily follows : if the hip is fixed, then the hip bone will prevent the trunk from being lowered too much. Ten dual movements to ten respirations. Be careful always to start exhalation in good time, perhaps a moment before the twist is complete.

The way here described of performing this exercise is the normal one. As a change, however, you may do it the opposite way, which give the muscles of the back more work and those of the abdomen a little less. You should begin as before by lifting the arms and turning the trunk, say, to the left (Fig. 22). But then instead of leaning "forward " (over the left hip), you lean *backward* over the right hip (Fig. 44), when a rightabout twist brings the chest downward (Fig. 43). Thereupon the upper body is raised and leaned " backward " over the left hip (Fig. 42), where a leftabout twist brings the chest downwards once more (Fig. 41). The breathing is now reversed, of course, so that you inhale during raising and backward-leaning, while the exhalation takes place with the twisting.

FOURTH DEGREE

This is an increase in strength of that in the Third Degree, described " normal way." Each time, during exhalation, when one slowly raises the body and leans over the opposite hip, one performs 4 to 8 jerky side-bendings (like the extra movement in Fourth Degree of Exercise No. 4). These " sidethrows " must of course be done in the waist, not in the shoulders.

EXERCISE No. 8

Bending and Stretching of the Arms, partly Loaded with the Weight of the Body

FIRST DEGREE

Stand facing a chest of drawers, the end of a bed or similar object with your feet about a yard from the same and heels together. If the distance be increased, the exercise will at once be more difficult to perform. Put your hands on the particular piece of furniture shoulder

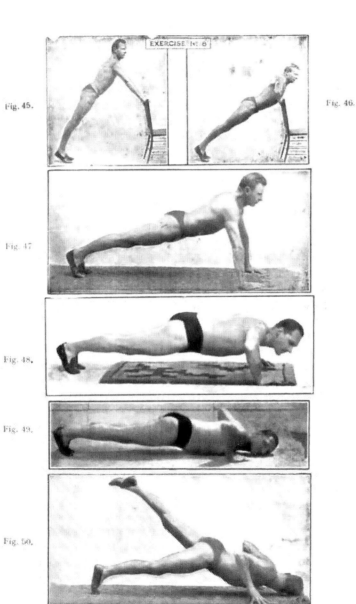

Fig. 45.

EXERCISE № 8

Fig. 46.

Fig. 47

Fig. 48.

Fig. 49.

Fig. 50.

F

distance apart (see Fig. 45). Then sink the body slowly forward by bending the arms, at the same time turning the finger-tips inwards and bringing the elbows well outward and slightly up (Fig. 46). This is done during inhalation. The body is held as straight as a plank and the heels are raised off the floor while the arms bend. While exhaling, the arms are slowly straightened again, and the fingers point once more to the front, heels lowered. Ten dual movements to ten respirations.

Every time the arms are being bent, you may turn the head slowly to one side alternately, bringing it back to the front on stretching the arms. A common mistake is to push the seat out backwards and bend in the hips. People with weak backs go to the other extreme by dropping the abdomen.

If for some reason or other only one arm can be used, stand a pace from the wall and put the arm straight out with palm against the wall, in height with one's head. Then bend and stretch the arm as before.

SECOND DEGREE

Resting on palms and knees on the floor. Carry out similar arm and head movements. The fingers are now constantly pointing inward 45°. You should inhale with the downward movement because the elbows are brought out to the sides and the chest thus opened, whereas in other exercises where the body is doubled up, you naturally exhale while bending forward or downward.

THIRD DEGREE

The normal way. On the floor, resting on palms and toes only (Fig. 47). To be sure that the body is kept straight, let a friend control you to begin with, or you can glance sideways into a mirror. If you find yourself either dropping or raising the seat before the exercise is finished, you had better drop on to the knees and continue in this position of the foregoing degree. Inhale while going down (Fig. 48), exhale coming up, and turn the head to alternate sides (Fig. 49).

FOURTH DEGREE

Either do the exercise on the finger-tips with hands spread out or lift each straight leg alternately on going down. These two advanced methods can, of course, also be combined (Fig. 50).

One can also perform the arm movements quicker; for example, bend and stretch twice during a deep inhalation and three times while exhaling. If you are very strong, you can put one hand on the back while moving up and down by the effort of the other one only. This hand should be well in under the body. Particularly use the weakest arm.

The Bath, as it may be arranged in houses without special bath-room

A simple plan is to use an ordinary tub and jug; the best and most practical thing, however, is to get a flat sponge-bath, a hand shower-bath and an ordinary bucket. The hand shower-bath is easily filled by dipping it in the full bucket. If you do not like absolutely cold water, which is only good for the nervous system so long as one does not suffer from "nerves," you should use lukewarm or warm water.

To all weak or nervous persons I would rather recommend a hot bath, perhaps finished by a short colder douche.

The bath itself can, of course, be taken in different ways. Some are in the habit of taking a large sponge, dipping it in the water, and squeezing it over themselves. I will describe the most practical mode of procedure.

Stand up in the middle of the " sponge-bath," and pour the contents of the sprinkler over yourself. Then sit down in the middle of the bath, and pour the rest of the water in the bucket over you. With a little practice you can manage so that the water divides and runs down the body, without any worth mentioning being spilt. But be careful not to make water-jets of your elbows. If it be absolutely necessary that not a drop shall be spilt, you should sit down straightaway, before beginning to wet yourself. But even if you are standing up, you need not upset more water than if you were sprinkling the floor for sweeping —and that is a good thing to do.

Then lie down on your back in the bath, which will cause the volume of water to rise, so that by rolling a little over on the sides you can get both arms and sides under water. Scoop the water up from the sides, first in one hand, then in the other, to get it up to the front parts of the body that the water cannot reach. Then sit up, well back in the bath, and pour water some few times down the sides of the chest, forming a cup with the two hands. Afterwards pour water in the same way over the upper and under side of the thighs, then bathe the seat, and finally stand up again and wash the lower part of the legs and the feet.

When once a week you have used warm water and soap, swill yourself all over afterwards with cold water, using a jug or hand shower-bath.

If you have got no tub at all you can still have a sort of bath by simply standing on a mat and slapping the body smartly all over with a towel dipped in cold or lukewarm water, or, in the event of only one towel being handy, by wetting the body with the hand.

Drying the Body

While still standing in the bath, wipe or rub yourself down a few times with the hands, with similar action to that described under Exercise 11, but of course you must also rub down the front of the legs. This will get rid of most of the water. In the same way wipe the water off the arms and hair, into the bath. Then shake the water from your feet, stand on a small rug or mat* and begin the actual drying of the body with a towel. First dry your hair, face, and neck, so that the water shall not drip from them on to your body whilst you are drying it. Next rub the front of the body several times up and down from the neck to the abdomen, and several times up and down the sides from the armpits to below the hips. The best way of doing this is to fold the

* If you use one and the same mat or carpet for all the exercises, you ought, while drying yourself, to have it double, with the wrong side up, and then when you have finished the exercises it should be hung out to dry.

towel double round the one open hand, while you hold both ends of it in the other hand (see Fig. 51).

Then comes the turn of the shoulders and the back. Fling the towel over the one shoulder, take hold of each end with one hand, and work up and down with both hands alternately, so that the back gets dried obliquely (see Fig. 52). But, at the same time, slide the towel along sideways, so that by degrees the back gets rubbed several times over from the edge of the one shoulder to the other and back again. Then pass the upper end of the towel over the head so that it now rests on the other shoulder, change hands (that is, the hand that was uppermost before should now be undermost) and repeat the process, the direction of the movement crossing the first in an X. Then let the top

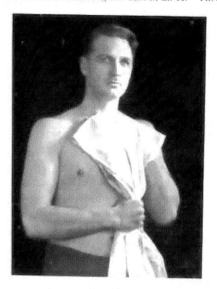

Fig. 51.

end of the towel slide down over the shoulder and arm, and alter your grasp of that end, so that the towel is now held as shown in Fig. 53. By now passing it quickly backwards and forwards, pulling with each hand alternately, nearly the whole of the back gets rubbed, from the loins up to as high as you can reach, and then in zigzag right down to the heels, and up again to the loins.

After this dry the hands and arms with the help of the movements described in Exercise 10 (the towel must of course be held between the open hand and the skin). If you have a tendency to cold arms—which is often the case with men who wear long-sleeved woollen vests, whereas women rarely feel the cold in their arms—they can be dried before the body. Then dry between the legs, and after that the fronts and sides

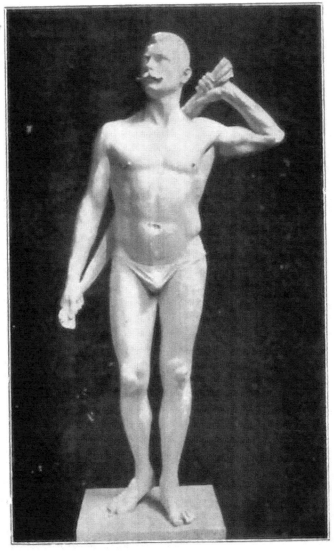

Fig. 52.

THE LIFE-SIZE STATUE OF THE AUTHOR
MADE BY THE DANISH SCULPTOR, BORGERBJERG

of the legs. Lastly dry the feet, first one, and then the other, and you should habituate yourself to doing this standing on one leg like a stork, which constitutes a very good *balancing exercise*. The soles of the feet are best dried by taking one end of the towel in each hand and pulling it towards you, with each hand alternately, and while you are drying between all the toes—there is plenty of time for that—rest your heel upon your knee. If you only set aside one quarter of an hour for

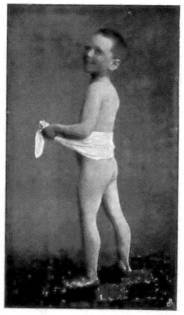

Fig. 53.

IB, THE AUTHOR'S ELDEST SON, AT THE AGE OF 4½ YEARS.

physical exercise, you must certainly not sit down upon a chair to rest during the time.

People who know how to dry themselves will perhaps consider these minute directions superfluous. Still, I have seen many stand and fiddle about with the towel for several minutes without getting properly dried even then. And I am thinking, too, of all the people who have, so to speak, never been in the position of requiring to dry themselves after a bath, because they have hardly ever done such a thing as to take one.

The Rubbing Exercises

General Remarks

I have ten composite rubbing exercises, to be performed in air-bath costume, during which the surface of the entire body gets thoroughly and systematically polished. The rubbing is done with the palms of the hands, and should be a simple stroking or friction to begin with ; later on, as one's strength increases, it should be so vigorous that it becomes a sort of massage, if not for the internal muscles further from the surface at any rate for the thousands of small muscles connected with the vessels of the skin, which are strengthened and developed more in this manner than by any other mode of procedure whatever.

After you have followed up my System for some time, the skin will assume quite a different character ; it will become firm and elastic, yet soft as velvet and free from pimples, blotches, spots, or other disfigurements. Many have recommended of late a revival of the custom of the ancient Greeks, viz. : that of performing physical exercises without clothing. Still one requires to be very much hardened—ordinary people could not possibly stand it at first—to do ordinary exercises in front of an open window during the cold seasons of the year. My rubbing exercises, on the contrary, can be carried out under such conditions, even by those most susceptible to cold. As a matter of fact, one keeps warmer, whilst doing them perfectly nude than when standing still with all one's clothes on. As a proof of this I may state that I can easily keep comfortably warm in the open air, even when it is freezing, or a cold wind is blowing, whilst I am going through my rubbing exercises, whereas I might sit and shiver driving in a carriage in the same weather with all my clothes and an overcoat on. This may sound strange, but it is nevertheless true. I can only say, " Try it yourself ! " The secret lies in the fact that a solid warmth is produced on the surface of the skin where it has been rubbed, even if only lightly, and this warmth lasts several minutes ; nor does it disappear whilst other parts of the body are being rubbed in their turn, so long as one proceeds according to a settled plan. The parts that might suffer most from cold receive in " My System " the most rubbing.

By performing " preliminary " movements to several of these exercises one learns how to move the body and legs and how to breathe during the performance. Not before this can be done quite automatically should the rubbing be added. To undress is therefore unnecessary during these " preliminary " movements. It is also recommended that persons susceptible to the cold should, during the colder parts of the year, wear some clothing while studying the book and trying the rubbing exercises themselves. Do not stand naked while reading in the book. Not before four to five complete rubbing exercises have been mastered is it safe to do them stripped without risking a cold or worse.

They are all performed standing, that the body may not get soiled or dusty again after the bath. As in addition to providing stroking of the entire surface of the skin they include a number of muscular exercises for the arms, shoulders, breast, and back, six leg exercises, two forward and backward bendings, two sideways bendings, and two trunk-twisting exercises (a slow and a quick one of each of these three main forms of trunk movements), they form a *complete whole in themselves* and can very advantageously be carried out in the evening, for instance, before going to bed, if you have done the first eight exercises with the bath in the morning. It is only a matter of 6 or 7 minutes. *It is advisable for ladies to stroke the front of the body in an upward direction, instead of from above downwards. This applies to Exercises 11 and 18* (see directions in " My System for Ladies").

The slow exercises—that is, those wherein the movements nearly synchronise with the natural, full respiration (Nos. 10, 11, 12, 13, 14 and 15)—are performed still more slowly by advanced persons as they by and by learn to breathe more deeply ; at the same time the actual stroking is increased in strength, or more elaborate rubbings are performed together with each breath. The quick exercises, however (Nos. 16, 17 and 18, and to a certain extent No. 9), are performed still faster, with the greatest possible number of movements during each respiration.

The limbs, on the whole, get stroked more *towards* the body than from the body, and it should also be remembered that more strength should be exerted when stroking in towards the trunk. It is a good plan at first to rub a little vaseline, lanoline, or something of the kind on the nipple of the breast, and if at all hairy into the roots of the hair as well. This precaution prevents smarting and irritation.

EXERCISE No. 9

Rubbing of Feet, top of Back, and round the Neck

Rest your right hand on the bedpost, a chair, or a door-handle, and rub with long powerful strokes the top and sides of one foot 25 times with the other foot, the sole of which thus of course itself gets rubbed (see Figs. 54-57). *At the same time* rub with the left hand the back of your neck as far as you can reach *from the top* down the middle of the back (Fig. 54), all round the neck (Figs. 55 and 56), and up and down the throat (Fig. 57). Then change about and begin the same number of rubbing movements with the opposite hand and foot. The whole exercise should last for eight full respirations. People who are inclined to get too much blood to the head, and cold feet, ought to perform this exercise at the end, after No. 18.

EXERCISE No. 10

Rubbing of Arms and round Shoulders, with full Knee-Bending

PRELIMINARY MOVEMENTS

A. Arm movements.—Either stand up or sit down. During inhalation move the arms as far backwards as possible, then slap them across the chest as shown in Fig. 58. During this last movement begin exhala-

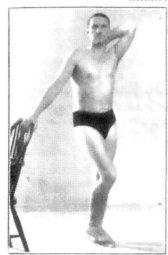

Fig. 54.

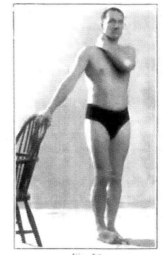

Fig. 56.

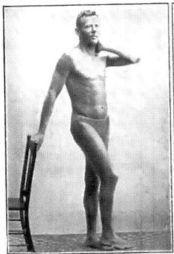

Fig. 55.

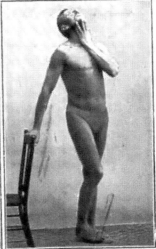

Fig. 57.

tion and continue same for a while after the arms have " crossed." Ten
repetitions to ten full respirations. Alternately put the left and right
arm uppermost. This exercise has from time immemorial been adopted
by cab drivers when on a cold morning they sit on their boxes awaiting
fares.

  B. *Knee-bending.*—Stand with your feet comfortably apart, arms
hanging by the sides, palms to the rear (Fig. 59). Lift the outstretched
arms slowly upwards with palms downwards until they reach shoulder
height (and shoulder distance apart) while inhaling. During the following exhalation perform these movements : bend the knees quickly until
the squatting position is reached without raising the heels, then return
sharply to the standing position while lowering the arms. If the arms
be lowered too soon one may easily fall backwards. People with weak
knees or a bad balance can support themselves by the end of a bed or
by a chair, and omit the arm movements. Ten complete movements
during ten respirations.

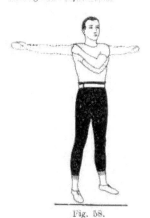 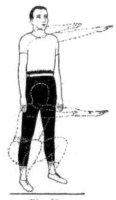

Fig. 58. Fig. 59.

THE RUBBING

  Extend the left arm, palm downwards. With the right palm.
stroke the upper side of the left arm (Fig. 60) from the tips of the fingers
to the shoulder and on up to the neck (Fig. 61)—then back again to the
finger-tips (Fig. 60)—after that, in the same way, the under-arm up to
the armpit (Fig. 62), and then inwards across over the left breast (Fig.
63) ; here the right hand relaxes its hold, immediately slapping the left
shoulder-blade smartly as far back as possible, *under* the left arm, which
at the same time is bent so that the left hand can take firm hold round
the right shoulder (Fig. 64). Then the right hand strokes the part from
the shoulder-blade in under the left armpit, when it relaxes its hold,
while the left hand has *at the same time* stroked the upper side of the
right arm from the shoulder bone (Fig. 65) down to the finger-tips.
The arms will now be stretched out in front of you once more, and the
movement is finished, the left hand resting meanwhile above the right,

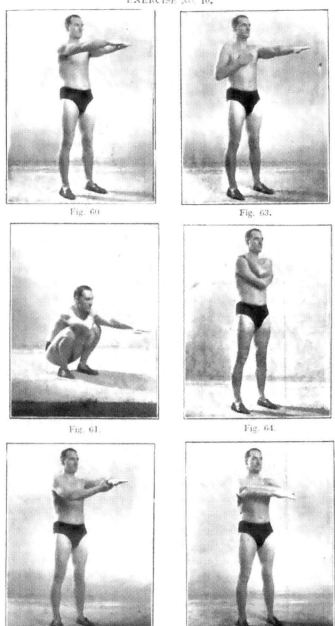

Fig. 60.

Fig. 63.

Fig. 61.

Fig. 64.

Fig 62.

Fig. 65.

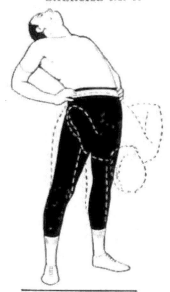

Fig. 66.

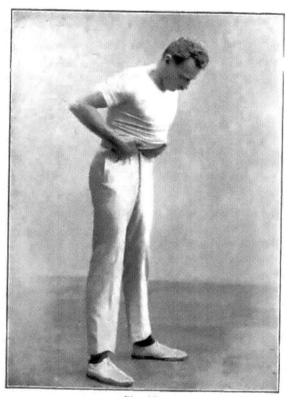

Fig. 67.

ready to begin an *absolutely corresponding* action (but replace the word " right " with " left," and vice versa, in the above description).

It will be seen that each complete movement falls into a measure of five beats which, with a very little practice, will proceed mechanically to your counting one, two, three, four, five. There should be ample time for ten of these movements of five beats, beginning with the right and the left hand alternately. When you have really learnt the exercise, do not count with each beat, but only each complete movement. Exhale during the first 2½ beats and inhale during the last 2½ beats, because it is natural to start inhalation at the moment you begin to open the arms just before they are slapped. A preliminary inhalation is taken while the arms are being raised slowly to the front before starting the exercise.

The outsides of the arms are rubbed considerably more than the insides, the skin on the back of the arms always needing it more ; after some time has elapsed, the arms and shoulders have grown firm and round and the skin feels like satin—with no roughness on the back of the upper arm, and no wrinkles at the elbow.

Not until after long practice, when one can take very full respirations, should two complete movements be performed during one respiration ; that is, five beats during inhalation and five whilst exhaling.

The rubbing is combined with the full-knee-bendings by sinking down simultaneously with the first beat (Fig. 61) and rising during the second. There are therefore no leg movements during the last three beats of each complete rubbing-movement.

EXERCISE No. 11

Full slow Backward and Forward Bending with Rubbings of Front and Back of Body lengthwise and Abdominal Movements

PRELIMINARY MOVEMENTS

A. Trunk bending.—Stand with feet apart and hands on hips. Bend the trunk and head slowly backward as far as possible, while inhaling (see Fig. 66). Then whilst exhaling bring the trunk forward and continue to bend it completely downward. Then rise and bend once more backwards, inhaling. Perform 20 such double movements with 20 full respirations.

The trunk is moved steadily without pausing at either end. During the forward-downward bending the muscles of the back and neck should relax, so that the weight of the trunk and head helps to " pull " downwards until you can look through your 'egs. The knees are bent as little as possible. Do not forget to begin the exhalation in time, so as to avoid holding the breath. If you feel dizzy at first you may support yourself with one hand.

B. Abdominal movements.—Lay the hands flat on the " stomach." Fill the lower part of the lungs with air till the abdominal wall is distended. Then empty again this portion of the lungs whilst pulling with the hands, so that the relaxed abdomen is pressed inwards and upwards under the ribs (Fig. 67). Twenty such " abdominal respirations" are to be performed. When after practice the abdominal muscles are stronger and under better control, the assistance of the hands may be dispensed with.

THE RUBBINGS

Every time the trunk has been bent backward (Fig. 68), stroke quickly downwards with the palms of the hands over the whole of the chest and abdomen, which should be well distended. Then when the trunk commences its forward movement, the abdomen is pulled in as much as possible, after which the hands are drawn apart (Fig. 69) and carried round to the small of the back as high up as is convenient (Fig. 70). With thumbs pointing downward, the rubbing is then continued over the loins, seat and back of the legs (Fig. 71) down to the ankles. The trunk is here bent as far downward as possible, with the back curved, and you then, without pausing, start to raise it again, the hands passing round the insteps and stroking up along the shins (Fig. 72), and the fronts of the thighs (Fig. 73), where the hands are taken off. Swing the body over backwards again, stroke once more down the chest (Fig. 68), and the combined movement which has just been described is repeated.

For women it is better not to take the hands away as they rise, but to stroke uninterruptedly from the instep up to the collar-bones, slipping the hands thence to the back as the forward movement begins (see " My System for Ladies ").

The various movements should glide evenly over into one another, and the strokes be long and continuous. Only on the small of the back should one rub up and down a few times when one has become able to breathe out more deeply, and hence have more time to perform such extra movements during the exhalation. Twenty complete combined movements are performed. Every other time, or else the last ten times, stroke up the inside of the legs instead of up their fronts. The knees may at first be bent a little during the forward bending ; later on the legs should be kept rigid all the time. Do not forget the special movements of the abdomen, which are highly beneficial to the intestines. This is the only exercise in the whole of " My System " where the abdomen should be drawn in, but then it is done as completely as possible, and for a few short moments only, in that it is quickly alternated with a full " blowing out " of the abdomen. By this means a powerful internal massage is given, which has just the opposite effect to that of a continuous indrawing of the abdomen, which is so harmful, owing to the fact that there is no internal massage or movement at all.

EXERCISE No. 12

Slow Trunk-Bending Sideways, with Half Knee-Bending and Rubbing upwards on Thighs and Hips and across the Abdomen

PRELIMINARY MOVEMENT

Stand with hands on hips, and feet wide apart. While exhaling deeply, bend the left knee, leaning the trunk at the same time sideways over the right leg, which must be kept quite straight. Then raise the

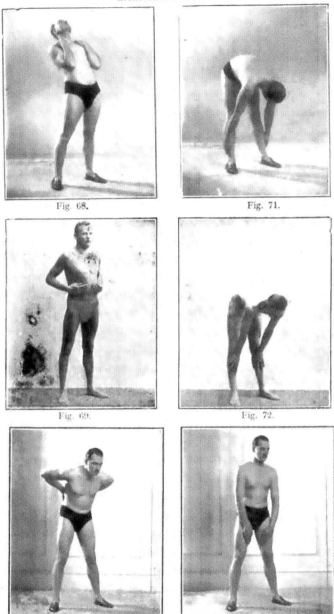

Fig. 68.

Fig. 71.

Fig. 69.

Fig. 72.

Fig. 70.

Fig. 73.

body slowly and resume the upright position with both legs straightened, at the same time inhaling. Remain thus for a moment, commencing exhalation, then lean the trunk sideways over the straight left leg, bending the right knee, while finishing the exhalation. Again rise whilst inhaling, stretching the right leg; pause in the upright position while commencing the exhalation, and for the second time bend over the right leg while completing it. Continue with intermittent pauses these swaying movements, making in all 12 trunk-bendings to the two sides alternately, during 12 complete respirations. Keep the face and breast to the front the whole time. It is a common fault to bend the trunk obliquely forward instead of sharply to the side. Remember, also, always to bend over the stretched leg; but the weight of the body should be thrown upon the bent leg, hence you should be able, in the correctly bent posture, to lift the foot of the stretched leg an inch from the floor and keep it there without losing the balance (see Fig. 74).

THE RUBBING

On bending to the left you place both palms firmly on the outer side of the left leg as far down as you can reach without bending forward (Fig. 75). Then while resuming the upright position, slide the palms upwards over the thigh, hip and half-way up the side of the trunk (Fig. 76). Here the left hand should be kept vertical under the right, which has been turned horizontal: the two forming the letter T. Now press hard across the abdomen with the hands still in the " T " position, the right " pulling " above the navel, the left " pushing " below it (Fig. 77). Having stroked right across the front (Fig. 78), the hands are taken off and then slapped down on the outer side of the right leg whilst bending the trunk to the right side and bending the left knee (Fig. 79), whereupon the whole movement is continued in the same way as described above, only with substitution of the word " right " for " left," and vice versa. Of course, the left hand is now uppermost (Fig. 80), and the stroking of the abdomen is now performed in the opposite direction. Beginners are prone to cross their hands when bringing them up from one of the legs, which, of course, is wrong: the hand which is undermost upon the leg should remain undermost also when moved across the abdomen.

Persons suffering from digestive troubles ought to relax or soften the abdominal muscles, so that the massage becomes as deep inwardly as possible. The same concerns persons with weak and distended abdominal wall. On the other hand, those with layers of fat on top of strong abdominal muscles should contract these (without holding the breath!) so that the superfluous fat gets squeezed between the palms and the hard muscles, and so loosens. In persons with a big " tummy," the abdomen ordinarily feels soft to the touch, both standing, sitting and lying. To ascertain whether the case is one of " distension " or just excessive fat, one lies flat on the back and lifts both straightened legs a few inches off the floor. Then feeling the stomach with the fingers, this part appears hard and swelling like a well-pumped football, or else you will find a flat muscular wall covered with soft fat. A distended thin abdominal wall will, of course, be strengthened and thickened by its possessor doing my exercises correctly; and will ultimately cease to give way to the pressure from the heavy bowels and liquid inside, and so

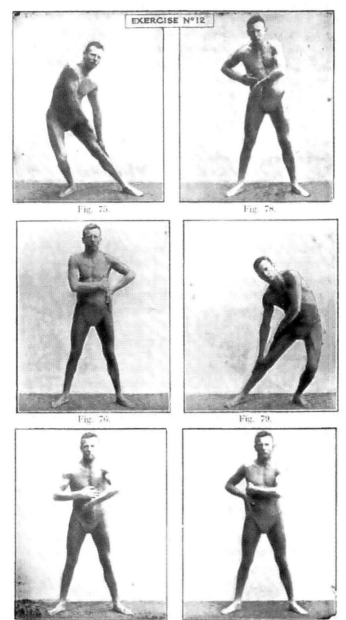

EXERCISE N° 12

Fig. 75.

Fig. 78.

Fig. 76.

Fig. 79.

Fig. 77.

Fig. 80.

loses its " tubby " appearance. But it is a wrong way to try and get
rid of it by keeping the abdomen indrawn.

When well advanced, one may perform the following extra rubbing
during each exhalation : as the lower hand has passed across the
abdomen, it continues in a large, complete circle upwards and then
across the chest (Fig. 81), of course against the direction of the stomach
stroke, then downwards, and finally once more across the abdomen.
Simultaneously the upper hand is swung round between the shoulder
blades (with palm outward), from where it, together with the forearm,
makes a long sweep down the back, and finishes across the seat (as is
also done in Exercise No. 15).

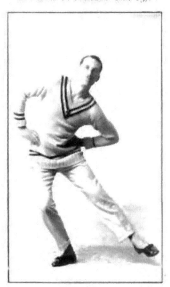 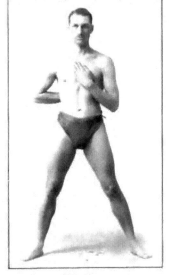

Fig. 74.   Fig. 81.

EXERCISE No. 13

Slow Trunk-Twistings to Alternate Sides, together with Rubbing vertically of Sides and Loins.

PRELIMINARY MOVEMENT

Sitting : In order to get the best results, i.e. suppleness in the waist,
it is a good plan to sit on a stool or chair with your back to a mirror.
Grip the chair legs with your feet and face the back of the chair. In
other words, sit astride. The seat must not move ! Whilst inhaling
fully, slowly twist to the left in the waist till you can look into the
mirror, with right arm across the abdomen, left arm in the hollow of the

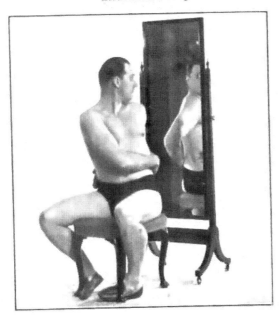

Fig. 82.

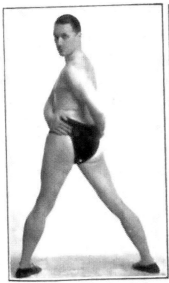

Fig. 83.

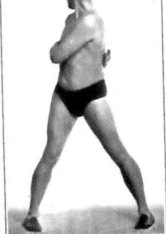

Fig. 84.

back (Fig. 82). Exhaling fully, twist slowly all the way round to the right, changing over the arms, and once again looking into the mirror. Go on thus, twisting left inhaling, and right exhaling for six full breaths. Return to front. Then do another six breaths, but this time twist to right inhaling, to left exhaling : twelve breaths in all.

Standing : Having done the above for a few days (or weeks, if you are very stout or stiff in the waist), you can do the movement standing as shown in Figs. 83 and 84. The feet must be very wide apart, toes turned inwards, and knees kept straight (braced back). This position, if maintained, will keep the hips still, and thus ensure that the twisting is done in the waist exclusively ! Carry on as above, twelve breaths in all, six each way.

THE RUBBINGS

The procedure is not quite the same now as during preliminary movement. The trunk only moves during the inhalations. Whilst exhaling, it remains twisted to alternate sides where the rubbing is performed.

Take up starting position : Standing, with feet very wide apart, toes in, knees straight ; your back to a mirror if handy. Arms hanging loosely at sides. Empty your lungs completely.

Whilst inhaling deeply, twist to the left in waist only, and bring arms to positions in Fig. 83. The left hand with palm outwards (as right hand in Fig. 84). During the whole of the exhalation massage up and down sides and loins moderately fast. The movement comes from the elbows ; but the wrists can also move. Fig. 83 shows the lowest position of the hands, Fig. 84 the highest. Again, inhale and slowly twist trunk completely round to the right (Fig. 84), changing over the arms whilst twisting. Now massage up and down as before, over sides and loins, till exhalation is finished. Then twist to the left inhaling, stop and rub again, exhaling. Carry on : twelve breaths in all.

This exercise reduces fat on hips and sides ; slims waist and makes it supple. Internal massage is also given to the liver and other organs. Later on you can increase the speed of the massage.

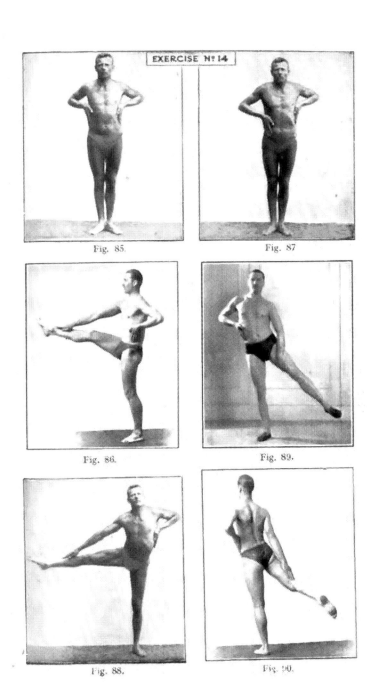

EXERCISE Nº 14

Fig. 85.

Fig. 87

Fig. 86.

Fig. 89.

Fig. 88.

Fig. 90.

EXERCISE No. 14

Slow Raising of Stretched Leg in three directions, with Rubbing up and down Leg and Lower parts of Trunk

PRELIMINARY MOVEMENT

Stand with feet almost together and parallel. Hands on hips, or still better to assist balance, with palms against flanks, fingers pointing downwards (Fig. 85). Slowly raise left leg forward as high up as possible, and lower it again, all the while inhaling. Repeat these movements with right leg, exhaling. Then raise left leg high up sideways to the left, and lower it again, inhaling ; and move the right leg in corresponding way while exhaling. Finally, raise the left leg backward as high up as possible and lower it slowly again, all during inhalation ; and perform the same movements with right leg during the exhalation.

The knees and ankles should be well stretched each time a leg is raised.

Repeat the whole performance twice more, and that will complete the exercise, the whole being three cycles, each of six double movements, and the performance will then last nine respirations.

Beginners who experience difficulty in keeping their balance can support themselves by gripping the back of a chair.

THE RUBBINGS

Starting position as Fig. 85, or with feet parallel. Leg movements and breathing exactly as in preliminary movement.

Each time a leg is raised forward, the corresponding palm should stroke down over the groin and out along the front of the thigh, the knee and the shin (Fig. 86), and while the leg is lowered, the palm strokes outward round the calf and then up the back of the leg, over the seat, and replaces itself upon the flank (Fig. 87). Each time a leg is moved sideways, the hip and outer side of the thigh are stroked (Fig. 88) during the raising of the leg, and when it is lowered, the palm strokes inward round the knee, back upon the inside of the thigh (Fig. 89), and over the groin to the flank. And each time a leg is raised backward and again lowered the palm strokes down over the loin, seat and back of the thigh (Fig. 90), then round the leg, upward on the front of the thigh, and back again to its starting position on the flank.

During all the raisings and lowerings of the leg the palm should continuously press hard against the movement of the leg. Eighteen double movements during nine respirations. Later, when you can take longer respirations, you may rub smartly up the abdomen and down the loins and seat in the last part of each expiration, this rubbing being very similar to that done in Exercise No. 18.

This exercise strengthens several muscles of the hips and lower back, which are otherwise seldom developed.

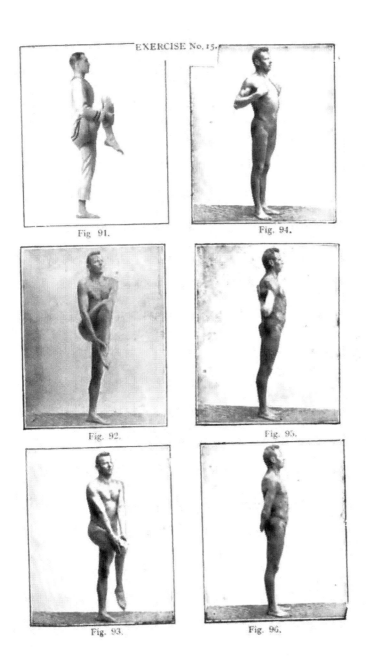

Fig. 91.

Fig. 94.

Fig. 92.

Fig. 95.

Fig. 93.

Fig. 96.

EXERCISE No. 15

Knee-Raising with Rubbing of Legs and Front and Back of Trunk lengthwise

PRELIMINARY MOVEMENT

Standing with feet almost together, lift one knee, grasp the shin with both hands and press the thigh against the body whilst leaning slightly backwards and inhaling (Fig. 91). Then let go the leg and resume the starting position ; pause for a second, then raise and grasp the other leg—all during exhalation. Then press and inhale as before. Perform ten such slow knee-raisings alternately with each leg during 10 full respirations. Should difficulty at first be experienced in balancing on one leg, then sit down on a chair, lean back and do the same movements.

THE RUBBING

Each time a knee has been lifted as far up towards the chest as possible without bending the body forward, you should take hold of the sides of the foot or the heel with both hands (Fig. 92). Then push the leg downwards (Fig. 93) and forward through the hands, thereby stroking it vigorously in an upward direction. When the leg is straight it returns to the other one while the hands continue their stroke upwards on the abdomen and the chest right up to the collar-bones, where they slip over to the sides (Fig. 94) and release their hold, the arms dropping loosely to the sides. Inhale during all this upward rubbing. During the following exhalation a short pause is enacted with the arms hanging down, and the other knee is lifted and the foot grasped. Thereupon perform a similar upward stroking of this leg and the front of the body during inhalation ; and so on. As the leg is lifted the toes should be the last to leave the ground ; thereby one is compelled to stretch the instep each time.

Whilst stroking the leg do not make a " short cut " and miss the knee—this is remedied by stretching the lower part of the leg well out before reaching the knee.

Later on the afore-mentioned pauses during the first and greater part of the exhalation are utilised by stroking lengthwise with the back of the hand down the back. The hand which corresponds with the lifted knee is flung up between the shoulder-blades (Fig. 95) and strokes downwards and across the loins and the seat (Fig. 96). You should also let the forearm take part in this stroke, pressing it well into the hollow of the back. As the exhalation after practice gets deeper, both arms are used after each leg movement, first the one, then the other, up to 4 times.

Persons with incipient varicose veins should perform the leg-stroking very carefully, and with more repetitions ; so that this undesirable complaint be " nipped in the bud."

Women who wish to obtain a firmer bust and slender hips should take one breast at a time, namely, the one over the lifted knee. And

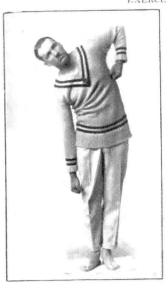

Fig. 97

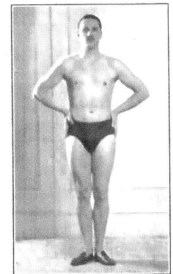

Fig. 98.

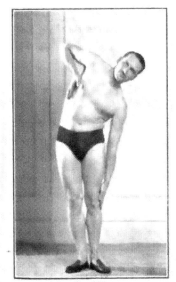

Fig 99

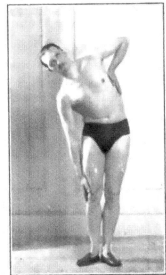

Fig. 100.

instead of the back-rubbing during exhalation, can now perform a zig-zag rubbing with the hands down the flanks and hips. One hand on each side, as illustrated in " My System for Ladies."

EXERCISE No. 16

Quick Sideways-Bending of Trunk, with Rubbing of sides of Trunk and Thighs

PRELIMINARY MOVEMENT

Stand with heels together, arms hanging down limp. Perform a number of alternate sideways-bendings, quickly and without the least pausing in the bent positions. You may also perform a sort of pumping movement with the arms, these being alternately bent and stretched downwards, as shown in Fig. 97. The exercise should last through four full respirations. One will in time be able to perform two double-movements (four "jerks") during inhalation, and the same number, or more, during exhalation. The neck must be stiff and the head kept erect and moving with the trunk, not bent separately as in Exercise No. 4, First Degree B.

THE RUBBING

Starting position : Hands flat against the hips, fingers pointing down (Fig. 98). Every time one bends to the left, the left palm strokes down the outer side of the thigh as far as the knee. Simultaneously the right palm is drawn up the right side as far as possible towards the armpit, the elbow being bent considerably, so that a longer stretch can be rubbed (Fig. 99). In a similar way the left hand strokes upward, the right downward, when the trunk is flung over to the right (Fig. 100).

Later on, as the pace of the movement increases, it must not be done at the expense of the force of the rubbing, or of the length of the movements. In other words, always press hard, and bend right over to the sides. It is of the greatest importance that the breath be not held, which so many persons are inclined to do when doing this and the two exercises following. It is a good general rule to move the trunk faster while exhaling, and slacken the speed somewhat during the inhalations.

EXERCISE No. 17

Quick Trunk-Twisting, with Rubbing across the Abdomen, the same way as the Twisting.

In all previous editions this exercise had the massage done across the chest—and against the movement of the trunk. Owing, however, to the fact that nearly everybody who learnt from the book did it wrong—some hopelessly so—I have now simplified the massage without in any way detracting from the exercise's effect on the trunk muscles and internal organs.

PRELIMINARY MOVEMENT

Sit, with hands on the hips, upon a stool, chair (astride, facing its back) or simply on the floor (with feet apart some 45 degrees) and grip your feet round the legs of the stool or chair, as shown in Fig. 101. Also face a mirror if handy. Unlike Fig. 101, start by sitting facing the mirror squarely with your shoulders.

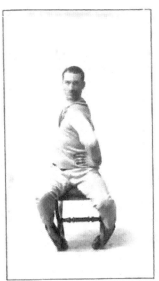

Fig. 101.

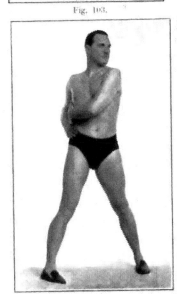

Fig. 103.

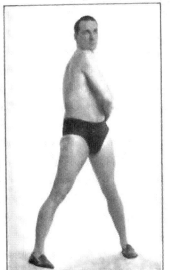

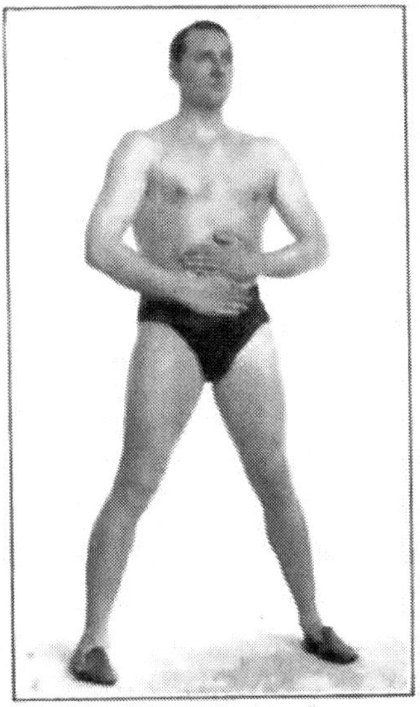

Fig. 102.

Fig. 104.

Then, keeping the head still, facing mirror—and this is important—twist the trunk to the left, simultaneously sliding the right hand to the stomach, the left to the middle of the back, and then twist completely round to the right, sliding the left hand to the stomach (a little farther than shown in Fig. 101), and the right hand to middle of back. Do this slowly a few times, keeping the head still, remember. Now do it to the proper deep breathing. Begin by twisting left, right to inhalation, and the same to exhalation. That is, two in and two out. Then have a go at two twists inhaling and four exhaling; and after a week or two try four in and six out, that is, ten twists to a breath. That should be enough in the preliminary stage. You can also try this preliminary movement, standing, with feet very wide apart, toes in, knees braced back, as shown in Figs. 102 to 104. Face a mirror as usual, and slide the hands round the waist in the relative "hips-firm" position. The object to aim at is to bring alternate shoulders under the chin and yet to keep head and hips facing the front. Do four full respirations a day.

The Rubbing

Stand, as shown in Fig. 103, facing a mirror (if handy), feet very wide apart, toes in, knees straight, and place the palms on the abdomen—one above the navel, the other below it.

Ultimately this exercise, like Nos. 16 and 18, is done at a very fast pace; but start slowly, like you probably did in the preliminary movement. Therefore, whilst inhaling deeply, twist left and massage from abdomen to left side of trunk horizontally (Fig. 102), then twist to the right, and rub across abdomen to right side (Fig. 104). Exhaling fully, do four twists with the same massage from side to side. Repeat, with special attention being paid to keeping head still to front, toes turned in, knees kept straight. *The hips must not move.* If they move a lot it means you are not supple enough—and—back on the chair you must go! The more the toes are turned inwards, the less likely you are of moving the hips, because of the inward twist given to both legs. Omitting to keep the head still leads to dizziness.

Having got used to six movements per breath, you can go on to ten : four inhaling, six exhaling. Stick to ten for a fortnight, then try six inhaling and eight exhaling. After that, it is a question of moving as fast as you can and breathing as deeply as possible. Eight inhaling and twelve exhaling—twenty per breath—is not impossible. My son, with his ten inches chest expansion, finds it possible. He is now 37 years old.

An inward pressure must be kept up by the hands all the time, as centrifugal force tends to move them away from the stomach when the speed is increased.

Fat men can massage over three different paths across the abdomen. And use them in successive strokes. The middle path, with one palm above, the other below the navel. The lower path, with both palms below the navel; and the upper, with both palms above it. This means a sort of ascending and descending zig-zag course. The more a "tummy" is worried, the quicker it will vanish.

Women should not perform this exercise. They have their own No. 17 in *My System for Ladies.* But one part of their exercise is the abdominal indrawing of Exercise No. 11, described in this book on page 93.

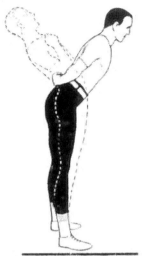

Fig. 105.

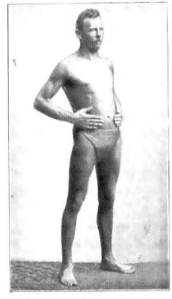

Fig. 106.

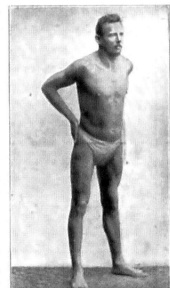

Fig. 107.

EXERCISE No. 18

Quick Backward-Forward Leaning of Trunk, with Rubbing Lengthwise of Front and Loins

In this exercise the trunk moves in the same directions as in Exercise No. 11, and this is the only resemblance.

Whereas No. 11 is a long slow movement, with indrawing of the abdomen, and bending of the neck, No. 18 is a short, fast movement, with stiff neck and back, and the abdomen pushed out all the time.

PRELIMINARY MOVEMENT

Stand with feet comfortably apart, and hands on the hips. Throw the trunk alternately backwards and forwards in short brisk swings without any pauses at all, nor any bending in the waist or curving of the back. The hips and abdomen are protruding on leaning the upper part of the body backwards ; and the seat is shot out on leaning forward.

As in the two preceding exercises, perform several double swings (from eight to sixteen " jerks ") during every respiration ; and let the exercise last four full respirations.

After a little practice you may in each backward movement thump once with both fists upon the chest, and in each forward movement upon the loins. The chest is struck by the inside, the loins by the thumb-end of the fists (Fig. 105).

THE RUBBING

Each time the trunk is flung backwards rub swiftly with both hands from below up over the abdomen, and with each hand on its respective side, outwards over the lower ribs (Fig. 106). They are then smartly brought round to the back, where they—while the trunk moves forwards—rub down over the loins and seat (Fig. 107). The back-rubbing is performed with the palms of the hands as in the longer stroke of Exercise No. 11. Whereas the back of the hands are used for the back-rubbing in Exercises Nos. 12, 13 and 15, where only one arm works at a time.

Ladies should make the front-stroke higher up, viz., from under the breasts up to the collar bones, as described in " My System for Ladies."

MY SPECIAL EXERCISES FOR THE NECK

These are not included in " My System " because they are not actually necessary to the health. But as it does appertain to physical beauty and a good appearance to have a well-developed neck, and as all the exercises for the neck which are to be found in other books of gymnastics only partially effect their object, and as, in the third place, it is only comparatively few who have an opportunity of going in for Græco-Roman wrestling, which brings the muscles of the neck and throat specially into play, I have appended a description of three exercises of mine for this purpose by the help of which a man or woman with a thin neck can make it strong, and ⅞in. more in circumference, in three months.

I no longer do these exercises myself, since by dint of practising them, my neck has already become too thick and therefore apparently too short. I wear an 18-inch stand-up collar, and if a man weighing twenty stone takes hold of me by the back of my head, I can lean my head back and, without using my arms, swing him right round with his feet in the air. My trick, " The suspended anvil," is also much more a test of the strength of the neck than that of the stomach, as I lie with the back of my head resting on one chair and my heels on another, while a couple of smiths with great sledge-hammers hammer away on an anvil weighing 200 lbs. placed directly upon my abdomen

1. Bending the head backwards and forwards

Bend the head well down to the front and grasp the upper part of the back of the head with both hands—fingers interlaced (see Fig. 108). Then, while bringing the head back, resist the movement by strong pressure with the hands. When the head has, however, slowly forced its way back, place your hands under the chin (see Fig. 109) and press to resist the bending forward of the head, and so on, backwards and forwards, from ten to fifty times

2. Bending the head to the sides

Lean the head over to the right and place the left hand against the temple as shown in Fig. 110. Then bend the head very slowly over to the left, pressing hard with the left hand in the contrary direction. When the head has come quite down to the left, take away the left hand and place the right hand against the right temple. The head then returns to the opposite side, the right arm resisting, and so on in alternate directions, from five to twenty-five times.

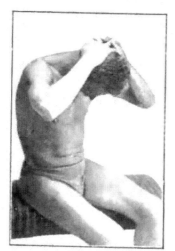

Fig. 108.

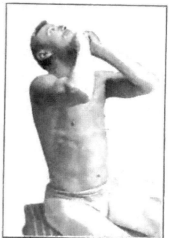

Fig. 109.

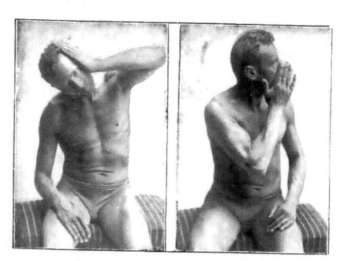

Fig. 110.

Fig. 111.

3. Turning of the head round to the sides

Turn the head to the left, place the right hand against the right jaw, as shown in Fig. 111.

Then turn the head slowly round to the right, resisting the movement by the force of the right arm. When the head is turned well to the right take away the right hand and place the left one against the left jaw, to oppose the head turning to the left, and go on thus five to twenty-five times, first to the one side, then to the other.

MY SPECIAL FOOT EXERCISES

ought to be done by all persons with a tendency to flatfootedness. The arch of the feet is also an important point as regards beauty, and even the most shapely foot is improved by a symmetrically arched instep. Besides which, my Foot Exercises are a never failing means of warming the feet in a few minutes. They may be performed at any time of the day, when you are sitting in a chair, or when lying in bed just before going to sleep.

FOOT EXERCISE No. 1.—Double-bending of the Feet

This exercise falls into a measure of four beats :—

1st Beat.—Bend the foot upwards at the ankle, as well as the toes, as much as possible. (See Fig. 112.)

2nd Beat.—Bend the toes downwards without moving the foot at the ankle. (See Fig. 113.)

3rd Beat.—Straighten the ankle while the toes are still bent downwards as much as possible. (See Fig. 114.)

4th Beat.—Bend the toes upwards, while the ankle is still held quite rigid. (See Fig. 115.)

To begin with, move one foot alone ; later on, both feet at the same time. When this exercise has been learned, do not count each beat, but only each complete movement, repeating the whole until you are tired

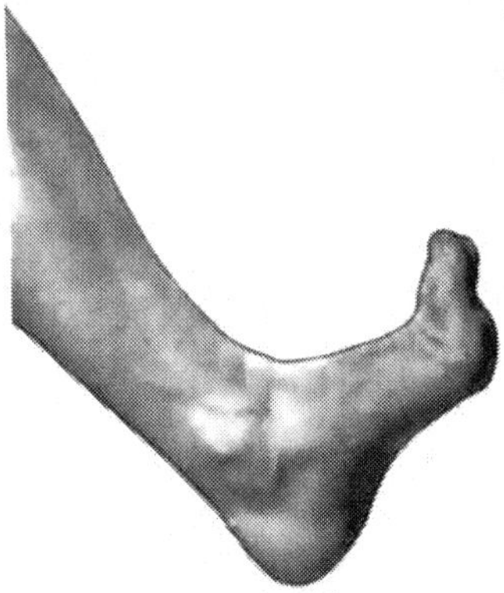

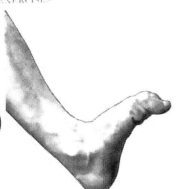

Fig. 112.
Bend the foot upwards at the
ankle, as well as the toes, as much
as possible.

Fig. 113.
Bend the toes downwards without
moving the foot at the ankle.

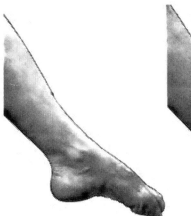

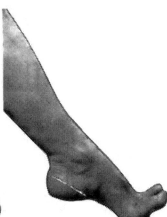

Fig. 114.
Straighten the ankle while the toes
are still bent as much as possible.

Fig. 115.
Bend the toes upwards while the
ankle is still held quite rigid.

FOOT EXERCISE No. 2.—Rotation of the Feet

While the leg is kept stationary, the foot only is moved round at the ankles, the great toe describing as wide circles as possible (Fig. 116), When tired, exercise the other foot in a precisely similar manner. When tired, exercise the first foot again, but in the opposite direction this time, following with the other foot in the same manner. You will soon learn to move both feet at once, and you may continue the exercise until tired without risk of hurting yourself.

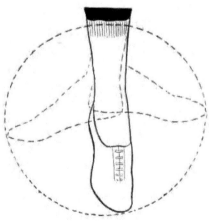

Fig. 116.

CONCLUSION

Dear Reader,

Whether you are weak or strong, young or old, I advise you to begin these exercises at once, and rather to-day than to-morrow. *But do not attack them too vigorously at first, unless you are accustomed to physical work.* Do not exercise for more than about ten minutes, following the programme given on page 52. Do not delay because you do not happen to have a bath ; you can buy one when convenient, and in the meantime be content to rub yourself all over with a wet towel. Later on, during your day's work, you will be surprised and delighted to feel the refreshing sensation pervading your body all the time. Here indeed we have an application of the proverb about small causes and great effects ! If you had spent a whole hour in Swedish drill, you would very likely have been more tired and disinclined for work than you used to be without any exercise whatever.

It is pure superstition to suppose that icy cold water is the only saving thing. The essential condition is that you should directly apply water, air, and rubbing to the entire surface of your skin, and that you should find it so pleasant that you feel a need and a desire to persevere. There will then come a time when you will use the water cold simply because it is more convenient, and no longer makes you shudder. And *then* it will make your nerves steadier still, although it might have had just the opposite effect, to begin with, on people with highly strung nervous systems.

Yes, it gives you a delightful feeling of satisfaction, having taken this early morning exercise and bath ! You get such a good conscience that even if later on in the day you have no time for any exercise or recreation whatever, it will not signify ; you may rest content, for you have indeed for this day *done* your duty to your bodily self.

* * * * * * *

Finally, have no fear that I propose to make a parody of a " strong man " out of you. I can well understand that you have a terror of getting to resemble those respectable gentlemen whose powerful physical development has proceeded in defiance of all laws of harmony and beauty. They feel called upon to round their elbows and to spread out and stick up their toes, to show how they can hardly walk for strength, and the greater the "dead weight" they can attain the better they are pleased. When they get photographed they lay themselves out to impress the beholder by forcing their unnaturally distended arm muscles into prominence, till they seem to be even more exaggeratedly developed and knotted than they are in reality ; or they lean forward with sombre mien and convulsively contract all the muscles in the front of their body. Every " strong man " magazine teems with repulsive pictures of the sort.

How supremely calm, how dignified and superior, and how delightfully harmonious, in comparison, the antique classical figures are ! In them you never see a muscle on the strain, unless this be called for in the position or movement represented. Everything bears the impress of perfect health and beauty : deep chest, broad and rounded shoulders, slender hips, the muscles of the trunk full, and the limbs substantial at the root, but growing gradually slenderer towards the delicate wrists and insteps. It is from this company that you should select your model.

It is *daily* physical exercise, if only for a short time, that has so excellent an effect. It ought therefore to become a *habit*, a necessity that a well-ordered household can just as ill dispense with as warm dishes for dinner or a cloth on the table. *Daily* exercise can by no means be replaced by, for example, one hour's gymnastics twice a week, or some hours' practice at games or sports in the week-end, however excellent the latter may be, regarded as supplementary.

Fifteen minutes every morning only come altogether to one and three quarter hours in the week; how can it be, then, that its effect on the human frame is so much greater and better? The reason is, you see, that during an hour's gymnastics in company a great deal of time is spent in changing one's clothes, in words of command, pauses, and in watching others ; in addition to which it is almost invariably the case that many of the exercises have comparatively little direct influence upon the health These seven short intervals of fifteen minutes, on the contrary, are, from the first second to the last, filled with hard work for the most vital organs. Finally, the body can only " digest " with advantage a certain amount of exercise at one time ; if it gets too much in one dose, the result may be more harmful than beneficial.

*   *   *   *   *   *

When, with such thoughts in my mind, I turn to physical exercises as they are taught in schools, it seems to me that these latter are anything but adequate. In my opinion, the instruction in this branch should assist the health and physical development, not only during school years, but later in life as well.

In most other subjects—reading, writing, and arithmetic, for instance—the pupil acquires knowledge of which he can make daily use in after-life. The physical instruction, on the other hand, requires rooms and apparatus which are not readily or daily accessible to him after he has left school.

In reality, there exist only two main forms of rational physical education for the young ; and each of these forms is supplementary to the other. Exercise in open-air sports and games constitutes the first of these methods, by which the physical and, to a high degree, the moral conditions of the young are simultaneously improved. The ideal, physically developed man must be, so to speak, a supple-limbed, agile being, whose chief characteristics are activity and power of endurance ; and these attributes are best attained through the medium of athletics and games, a method, to be sure, not calculated to produce that ponderous muscularity as artificially developed by exercises performed with heavy weights and with various kinds of gymnastic apparatus. But such a condition is not even worth the striving for, for where practical life is concerned, such can only be regarded as a dead burden, unwieldy, superfluous, troublesome, and probably unhealthy. Moreover, athletics and games have the further advantage of being, at the present day, the only means of encouraging in youth such mental qualities and attributes of character as courage, resolution, presence of mind, sense of honour, feeling of good fellowship, and readiness to assist the weak.

The second main form of physical culture for the young is the prosecution of a system of home gymnastics dealing with the vital organs of the body, and it must be a task of the school to make the children entrusted to its care skilful in the same and to urge them to the exercise of it.

The system must be so compiled that its use shall—in so far as it lies within human power—guarantee the maintenance of health and act as a safeguard against the majority of illnesses. The exercises, therefore, must principally and particularly have as object the promotion of the proper functional activity of the respiratory organs, the circulation, the skin, and the organs of digestion. A satisfactory development of the muscular system will result as a matter of course.

This ideal system must be *indissolubly connected with a daily bath, and self-massage*, but beyond that should require no apparatus whatsoever. Above all, it should be a system which the pupils can carry out in whatsoever conditions they may encounter in after-life. The pupils must not only learn the exercises themselves in school ; it must be impressed upon them that this little system must form and always remain a part of their morning (or evening) toilet. It must be capable of being performed with like benefit by the poorest as by the richest, by the weakling as by the athlete, by young and old, girls and boys, men and women. Its performance should not require more time than fifteen minutes daily, and, so as not to tax the memory, every single exercise must be such that it can be performed in exact repetition throughout life. Likewise all the exercises must be the same for all ; but, that they may be suited to different individuals, according to age, sex, or strength, each single exercise must be arranged in a number of different degrees of difficulty, *i.e.*, easier and more difficult ways of being performed.

Public schools, grammar schools, and high schools, as well as council schools, would be in a position to develop in their pupils, to a much greater extent than is now the case, a sense of the importance of personal hygiene and the proper care of the body, if through such a short system of home exercises—mine or some other—combined daily with bath and rubbing, they accustom them to the comforts of cleanliness and properly cared-for bodies.

A scholar who has had a physical education of this sort will really have brought out of his school experience something that will be of benefit to him through his whole life. This is the more desirable since the greater part of the physical and mental work of to-day is carried out under injurious external conditions. I am persuaded that the future will see my opinions put into practice.

* * * * *

Even if you are as fit and well as you think you can be, you ought all the same to accustom yourself to a daily bath and all-round daily exercise. If you are really fortunate enough to enjoy good health, you ought to put yourself to this slight inconvenience in order to retain and increase the same, but it is only the first step that is possibly a trifle unpleasant. You will soon get so " addicted " to these rejuvenating few minutes that you would not be deprived of them at any price.

You ought to do it, not for your own sake only, but even more for the sake of your descendants, that they may not degenerate through you.

How many children of healthy parents one sees come from the

country into the town and get completely absorbed by intellectual and commercial interests. If they are " fortunate " enough to become rich, they are soon involved in a whirl of social functions, high living, and all sorts of luxury. They then come to look with contempt on the manual labour that was the source of their parents' health and strength and to which they owe it entirely that their own health is not quickly wrecked by their one-sided intellectual overculture. But their offspring even in the first generation are delicate and overstrung, while their grandchildren stand with one foot in the grave when they are born, or at any rate, come into the world with a ticket of admission to the lunatic asylum. And all this misery might have been avoided had they reflected in time that the body is not a mere covering, of itself of no account for the soul and mind, but is the soil wherein all germinating power has its birth. So you must not impoverish your body, like a careless man farming rented land, but you should, like a prudent landowner, make it an object of wise and careful culture, remembering that this is an investment which yields good interest.

* * * * * * *

A body which is not daily exercised in every part, inside and out, decays, that is to say, grows decrepit and " old " before its time. There is, of course, no pleasure or advantage in growing old in years, if you are broken down, stiff, infirm, and full of ailments, with your intelligence well-nigh extinguished and your interests fled. Thus it is with no small number of people who have grown old because of the fact that they have their whole life long pooh-poohed *fresh air, sunlight, water and exercise.* The daily sight of these old wrecks has even given many young people a distaste for old age, so that they do not care in the least to do anything which will make them *live long.* One thus overlooks the fact that it is possible and indeed quite natural to preserve both the physical and the mental faculties almost unimpaired for at least a hundred years, and that this will mean an enormous addition to the happiness and wealth—both in money and experience—of the family, the race, and the State.

The chief advantage of rational physical exercise is thus not so much that the muscles and sinews grow stronger, as that all the internal organs, including even the brain, heart, and spinal cord, are daily cleansed in a rejuvenating bath. Do you think that a vertebral column, for instance, which is daily submitted to as many stretchings, bendings, and twistings to its utmost capacity, as is the case in "My System," can get stiff and calcinated and possibly impede the efficiency of the chief nerve-fibres which pass through it ? Or that the many deep-breathing exercises will allow the lungs, heart and arteries to lose their elasticity ? This is so far from being the case that even you, dear Sir, who are already getting on in years, if you will only begin these exercises now, will be able to grow more supple, and more erect and agile, than you were as a youth ; indeed, you will probably in a few months add a whole inch to your stature, as many others write to me that they have done. For this reason I would ask everyone who begins " My System " to have his height accurately measured, and likewise to measure the circumference of his chest, while the lungs are filled with air, and afterwards again when all the air has been exhaled. They can then see what the difference in the two chest measurements is after a space of six months.

Manufactured by Amazon.ca
Bolton, ON

37876599R00066